THE
G
PLAN
DIET

This book is for anyone and everyone who yearns for food freedom, a flatter tummy and glowing health from the inside out.

An Hachette UK Company
www.hachette.co.uk

First published in Great Britain in 2017 by Aster, a division of Octopus Publishing Group Ltd
Carmelite House, 50 Victoria Embankment
London EC4Y 0DZ
www.octopusbooks.co.uk
This edition published in 2018

ISBN 978-1-91202-375-2

A CIP catalogue record for this book is available from the British Library.

Printed and bound in China

10 9 8 7 6 5 4 3 2 1

All reasonable care has been taken in the preparation of this book but the information it contains is not intended to take the place of treatment by a qualified medical practitioner.

Before making any changes in your health regime, always consult a doctor. While all the therapies detailed in this book are completely safe if done correctly, you must seek professional advice if you are in any doubt about any medical condition. Any application of the ideas and information contained in this book is at the reader's sole discretion and risk.

Recipes marked 🍲 can be batch-cooked and kept for later in the plan. Ingredients marked * should be left out of the recipe if your digestion is particularly sensitive.

Special photography by Adrian Lawrence. Additional picture acknowledgements: **123RF.com** bizoon 23; Ekaterina Kondratova 101; Jean-Paul Chassenet 27; Kasto 125; Tanwa Na Thalang 126. **Alamy Stock Photo** Christoph Hermann 22. **Dreamstime.com** Robert Cocquyt 11. **Getty Images** Photography Ana Slavova 13. **Octopus Publishing Group** Lis Parsons 71; William Reavell 92.

Consultant publisher Kate Adams
Senior editor Pauline Bache
Copy-editor Jo Smith
Senior designer Jaz Bahra
Designer Megan van Staden
Production manager Caroline Alberti

THE G PLAN DIET

the revolutionary diet for
**gut-healthy weight loss
21-Day Plan & 75 recipes**

**AMANDA
HAMILTON
& HANNAH
EBELTHITE**

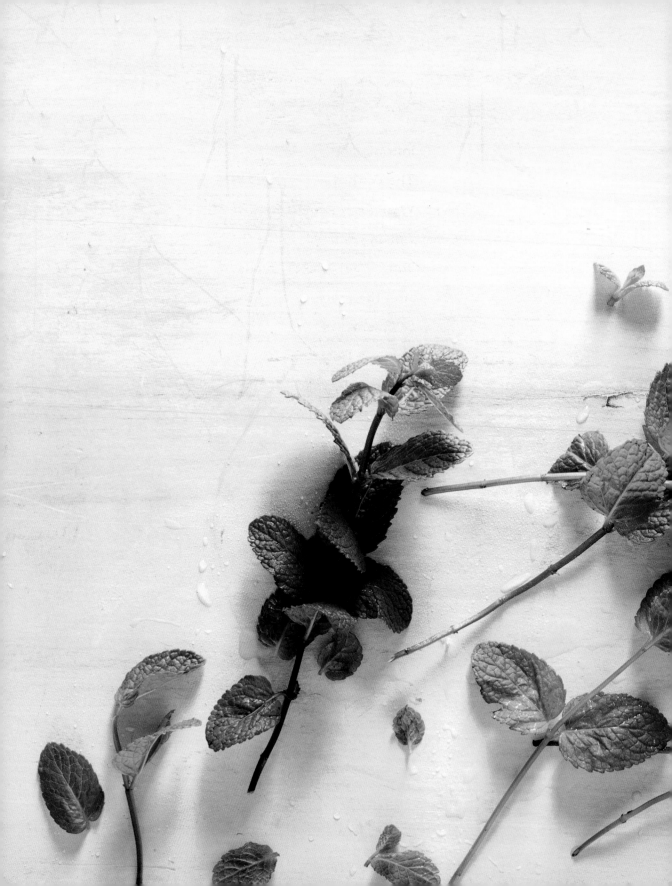

CONTENTS

INTRODUCTION

AMANDA SAYS

Let's face it, the gut is a hard sell. You can't see it, you've probably never given it much thought... And yet, it is probably the most exciting subject in health right now. We're seeing so many breakthroughs in our understanding of how the gut works, why it's important and what it means for the future of medicine. But this book isn't a dry dissection of all the research. It's the practical application. What can *you* do *now* to start benefitting from the latest findings? It's all in these pages.

The trillions of microbes in your gut are not only essential for digesting food, they also provide vital enzymes and vitamins, and control the calories you absorb, linking the health of the gut directly to weight issues. Whether you want to lose weight or not, or whether you're one of the one in four people who struggles with a digestive issue, you can benefit. The evidence is there, as you'll learn in the following chapters, that good gut health has an impact on your digestion, your day-to-day comfort and energy levels, your immunity, mental wellbeing and your chronic disease risk.

Even more exciting is the fact that *you* are in charge. What you eat determines your personal pick 'n' mix of gut bacteria that are then able to help keep you happy, healthy and naturally slim.

I wasn't always so enamoured with what lay beneath my navel. I took the well-trodden path of irritable bowel syndrome (IBS) and poor skin in my teens. The antibiotics that I took to improve the skin worsened the tummy troubles. My calorie-controlled diet – a rite of passage at that time – was a disaster for my gut and fed my cravings for carbohydrates.

It wasn't until I began to study nutrition that a change of diet solved the triple whammy of woes and changed my life, body and career forever. Fifteen years later I now understand and appreciate that my personal experience helped carve out what I now call my Rest, Re-wild and Rebalance approach to the gut.

The Rest phase is more like a detox. The D-word is often misconstrued but my meaning is lightening the load on the body, eliminating trigger and troublesome foods,

and supporting the organs of detoxification and elimination. I have run detox retreats for more than a decade using a fasting-style approach and the results after a few days alone are often astonishing. The version in this plan is less extreme – there's plenty of food – but your digestion will still benefit from a well-earned rest.

Then comes Re-wild. It might sound a bit 'hunter gatherer' but it requires no survival skills other than some online shopping for diverse and helpful ingredients, none of which are overly obscure or expensive.

Last but certainly not least, Rebalance is about getting to the place where you can easily maintain your well-deserved results, enjoy more freedom around food and, most important of all, feel happy.

So, please ditch the idea that being healthy from the inside out means living with endless restrictions or boring and bland food choices. Once your gut is healthy, a varied and inclusive diet is firmly back on the menu. For me that includes some delicious dark chocolate, a morning coffee or two, an occasional glass of wine with dinner or a gin and tonic with the girls. How very refreshing!

HANNAH SAYS

This is a book for anyone who wants a new approach to eating, to finally shift the excess and find their happy weight. It's for you if you're sick of trying diets that feel hard to follow and instinctively unhealthy. If your energy levels and mood are low but you feel powerless to raise them. If you feel your waist measurement is increasing, your shape is changing and you're not sure why. And if you'd like to be less reliant on processed foods and sugars but you're not sure how.

It's been a selfish endeavour, because it's really a book for me. On my 40th birthday, I resigned myself to never losing that extra half stone. My expanding waist felt like an inevitable consequence of creeping middle age. I love exercise but it no longer changed my shape.

I was a classic example of the busy person who thinks they don't have time to be healthier. I made sure my kids ate well, but would have their toast-crust leftovers for breakfast. I'd skip lunch or buy a sandwich, far too 'busy and important' to stop work and make something nutritious. Then I'd wonder why I could barely keep my eyes open come mid-afternoon. My skin wasn't great, my focus was lacking and my stomach was bloated. My doctor checked if it was a thyroid problem or peri-menopause. When it wasn't, I concluded it must be modern life.

As a health writer I've seen just about every diet trend come and go. I've tried many of them, in the interests of journalism, and I know a fad when I see one. Gut health is definitely a trend but it's no fad. It's an area of health that's here to stay.

So when Amanda and I started working on this book, I immediately volunteered to be its guinea pig. If I could stick to her plan and make it work, it could work for anyone.

In just a few weeks it genuinely changed the way I eat, for good. I've lost the taste for sugar, I bypass processed, convenience foods and prepare nearly everything from scratch. I've not been hungry. How have I fitted it into my oh-so-busy life? Erm, pretty easily. I can only think I was kidding myself that I didn't have the time.

By the end of the 21 days I was feeling lighter in weight as well as in mood. My usual 10 days of deranged premenstrual doom didn't happen. People remarked that I looked well and slimmer. I lost 3.6kg (8lb), at least 2.5cm (1 inch) each from my arms, thighs and hips and 7.5cm (3 inches) from my waist. Delighted is an understatement. As I write this, a couple of months on, I'm still enjoying the G Plan way of eating and I haven't regained any weight or inches. I really feel great.

And I know that you can, too. If you have any reservations about sticking to an eating plan, put them to one side and just go for it. It's only 21 days – that's shorter than any commitment you might make for Lent or 'Dry January' or the like. It works because it goes beyond what you can control and starts changing your body on a biological level. It's 21 days that can transform your eating, your shape and your life.

Gut. It's not a very attractive word, is it? We tend not to talk much about our gut. We probably don't think about it enough, either. Until fairly recently, even scientists were in the dark about the gut's importance in the body. Now they can't stop talking about it.

Much of the latest research is pointing to digestive health as not only the key to overall health, but the secret to losing weight and feeling fantastic – it's pretty exciting stuff. So it's time we all got better acquainted with what goes on down there.

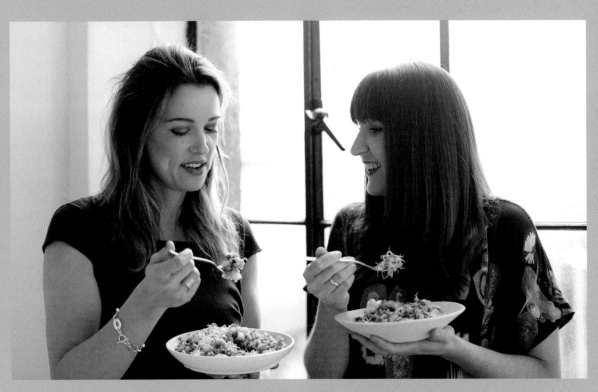

THE G WORD

You are more bacteria than human

There are 100 trillion microbes, mostly bacteria, living in and on your body. You are a walking bacteria colony. Bacteria outnumber your own body cells by about 10:1. And their genes outnumber your own genes by over 100:1.

Some bacteria reside on your skin, in your mouth and on the genitals. But the majority have set up home in your large intestine, the lower part of your gut, where they weigh a hefty 1.3kg (3lb). The bacteria are known as your microbiota and, collectively, they form your microbiome.

Now this might sound worrying. In the past, we've thought of microbes either as harmless parasites or dangerous pathogens. What with antibiotics, antibacterial wipes, cleaning products and hand gels, you'd be forgiven for thinking the goal was to wipe out all traces of bacteria from our lives. But the truth is we're nothing without them. We're still identifying all the hundreds, if not thousands, of strains that each have a role in looking after our health.

Where does the microbiome come from?

As babies we are born sterile and pick up our mother's microbiome as we pass through the birth canal during delivery. Babies who are delivered by caesarean section therefore have a more limited microbiome which is made up of bacteria from their mother's skin and the hospital, rather than the vaginal and faecal bacteria passed on during natural birth. The next major donor is breast milk and, again, babies fed on formula milk will have a different and more limited microbiome.

By the age of two we have a mature microbiome although it's always in flux and is moderated by diet – as we shall learn – lifestyle, stress, medication and even factors like owning a pet. Research has found children who grow up with a family dog share some of its microbes and may have a bolstered immunity overall from contact with their pet.

Studies also show people born by caesarean section, raised on formula milk and given antibiotics early in life are more likely to gain weight later on. But forget blaming your mum – or worrying about your kids – if you tick those boxes. That's in the past, it can't be changed and was the right choice for you or your parents at the time. You *can* change what happens to your microbiome in the future, and this book puts that power in your hands.

What does your microbiome do for you?

What *doesn't* it do would be a better question. Your healthy bacteria help you to digest food, protect you against pathogens, provide essential nutrients, enzymes and hormones and train your immune system. Your gut has the largest number of immune cells and the largest number of hormonal/endocrine cells in the body.

It's only been in the past ten years that we have had the knowledge and technology – called rapid gene-sequencing techniques – to enable us to identify different strains of bacteria and what their function might be.

Everyone's microbiome is unique, like a fingerprint. The interactions between microbes are complex and there's much we've yet to learn. But what the scientific world is increasingly discovering is that if there's something wrong with your microbiome, there will be something wrong with you.

The brain-gut axis

These days, you'll often hear the gut talked about in wondrous terms as our 'hidden brain', or 'silent voice'. That's due to something called the brain-gut axis and the fact that these two organs are far more closely connected than you might imagine. There are 500 million nerve cells in the gut – the largest number outside the brain and spinal cord. Together they're incredibly powerful.

It explains age-old terms like 'gut instinct', 'gut wrenching', 'gut reaction' or feeling 'gutted'; all those expressions that convey how our digestive system and our emotions are inextricably linked.

We understand that our feelings can affect our digestion – everything from butterflies in the stomach, to trips to the loo before an exam, to IBS when we're under stress. But we now know the brain-gut axis works both ways and stimulation of the gut can activate circuits in the brain.

Not just digestion

Think of your microbiome as your greatest health ally. If it's in balance you'll experience healthy digestion, high energy, fewer illnesses, good mood and clear thinking. If it's out of balance then digestive issues, low mood and low immunity can result. But it's even more important than that.

Research has found links between poor gut flora and IBS, inflammatory bowel disease (IBD), type 2 diabetes, Parkinson's disease, Alzheimer's disease, arthritis, cardiovascular disease, colon cancer, depression, anxiety, autism, asthma, allergies and respiratory tract infections.

It's unlikely to be a straightforward cause-and-effect situation – humans are more complicated than that. But many scientists believe it's more than an association: a poor microbiome can actually cause disease and influence behaviour and emotions. Germ-free mice (born into and kept in a sterile bubble) grow up exhibiting marked changes in memory, learning and emotions, and have an exaggerated stress response and autistic-like traits. Without bacteria, their brains don't develop normally.

The missing link when it comes to weight?

One of the key areas of gut research is focusing on weight loss. Studies in obese and lean sets of twins have shown that lean twins have a vibrant and diverse microbe community, while obese twins have far fewer useful microbes.

Gut microbes are involved in metabolism. They can alter the way we store fat, how we balance our blood glucose levels and how we respond to hormones signalling hunger and satiety. Having the wrong mix of microbes might set us along the path to obesity and type 2 diabetes.

Animal studies have shown that when sterile mice had microbes from an obese person or a lean person introduced into their intestines, those who received the obese person's microbes went on to gain weight and fat, while the mice receiving the lean's person's microbes didn't. This can also be reversed – the researchers transplanted the lean mice's microbes into the obese mice and they become a normal weight again. The potential for an 'obesity cure' in humans here is quite intriguing. Thankfully, we have the know-how to start nourishing the microbiome in a slightly less intrusive way.

FMT, the hard-to-stomach solution

If you're eating while reading this, you may want to put your food down for a moment.

The treatment these mice received was a version of faecal microbiota transplantation, otherwise known as FMT. And it could be the future of medicine. Essentially, it involves taking a stool sample from a healthy person and transferring the microbes into the gastrointestinal tract of someone who might benefit. Yes, it's a poo transplant.

In a world where antibiotic resistance is an increasing threat, you might just need to put your squeamishness aside and watch with interest. FMT is already in use and it can be a life-saving intervention. *Clostridium difficile* (or *C.diff*) is a potentially fatal hospital infection, picked up by patients who've had their microbiome all but wiped out by antibiotics. It can be very hard to treat... *unless* you transplant a healthy person's microbes into the patient, when an almost instant recovery can be seen.

So, it has a role in treating infection and it seems to work in mice. Could FMT be the next big slimming solution for us?

It's not unthinkable that Harley Street clinics will start offering it to the rich, overweight and curious (in the form of pills and suppositories, all very clean and clinical). But it would certainly be a speculative treatment at this stage. Before then, there's lots you can do to kick-start your weight loss. And it all starts with giving your gut – and those trillions of bacteria – a little more love and respect.

The future

Alongside FMT, probiotics (foods, drinks and supplements that contain live microbe cultures) are likely to become personalized and targeted. If disease can be identified by which microbes are present or missing in our microbiome, it follows that scientists may be able to produce probiotic strains that interact to bring the microbiome back into balance. Rather than broad-spectrum health supplements, we could see specific functional foods or pills designed to reduce or eradicate certain conditions.

There's also much buzz around the field of 'psychobiotics'. Not the title of a Hollywood blockbuster, but a term used to describe the potential for probiotics to address mental health conditions. A pill to reduce anxiety or a new form of antidepressant – amazing, yet not too far away perhaps?

Now: your health in your hands

In the meantime, we are far from powerless. The promising news is that the microbiome can change and adapt very quickly. The average lifespan of a microbe is just 20 minutes. Your microbes' genes change constantly in response to the food you give them. That's why humans all over the world are able to survive on vastly different diets.

It's also why people who restrict themselves to foods our prehistoric ancestors ate ('Paleo dieters') are ill-informed. Our own genes might take thousands of years to evolve but when it comes to food, our microbes are in charge and they're very accommodating. Eat a mainly meat diet and you'll develop the microbes you need to digest meat. Turn vegetarian and you'll lose them in favour of plant-digesting microbes.

But just because you *can* eat whatever you like, doesn't mean you *should*. The greater the amount of good bacteria you have and the greater its variety, the better. So how do we increase our own diversity?

What your microbiome dislikes

We know our microbiome isn't keen on the following things, so we should aim to avoid them as much as possible.

STRESS

When our bodies are in a low-level fight or flight response on a long-term basis, it's almost always felt in our digestion (thanks to that gut-brain axis). Stress has been linked to IBD, IBS, peptic ulcers, reflux, allergies and more. Scientists have shown that being under stress reduces the number and diversity of the microbiota.[1] And poor gut health, in turn, can cause or exacerbate mental health symptoms.

It can be hard to avoid, of course, and we often don't know how much stress is affecting us until we emerge the other side. But given the negative effect it can have on our gut, it's worth building some anti-stress practices into daily life. Meditation, yoga, exercise and spending time outdoors in nature are all well-tested techniques. Amanda swears by her favourite antidote to stress, her Labrador, Annie. But short of running out and buying a puppy, anything that carves some time out for you – be it reading a novel, singing in a choir, or playing in the shed with power tools – is a worthwhile investment in good gut health.

INACTIVITY

Exercise is a vital part of life and any weight loss efforts. A recent Irish study compared athletes and inactive people and found the former had a much greater variety of gut bacteria.[2] Other US studies confirm this, finding that exercise increases levels of butyrate, a compound produced by gut bacteria which supports immunity and may protect against colon cancer. Further research in Spain found a four-fold increase in immune-boosting bacteria strains in those who exercised.[3]

The World Health Organization suggests we each do 150 minutes of moderate-intensity exercise each week for good health.[4] That's at least five sessions of 30 minutes each, where you're active enough to be slightly out of breath and breaking a sweat. It also recommends two sessions a week of strength training. If you want the gains to exceed general health and move into increased fitness and better shape, we'd suggest having this as your absolute bare minimum.

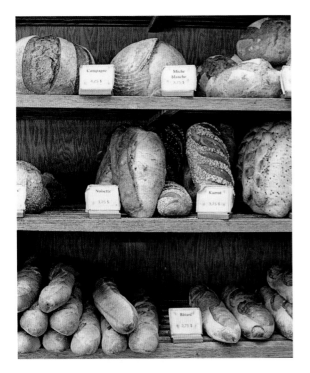

A PROCESSED AND LIMITED DIET

It'll come as no surprise that excess sugar isn't good for the gut. It suppresses beneficial bacteria and can allow unhealthy microbes to take over. A modern-day demon thanks to its prevalence in today's diets, sugar is linked with obesity and diabetes as well as poor skin and fluctuating energy levels.

Processed foods do our gut no favours. Very often high in sugar, salt, saturated or trans fats, additives and preservatives, they're also much lower on the nutritional scale than unprocessed foods. Refined, starchy carbohydrates, such as white flour, bread, pasta and rice, offer much less for the microbiome than their wholegrain alternatives. Avoid them and you automatically avoid foods like pastries, cakes and biscuits. Takeaways and ready meals are usually similarly low in nutrients and high in fat and sugar.

What your microbiome likes

The G Plan can help you to cut back on the things above and focus on those below, as it promotes a diet and lifestyle that's abundant in what your gut loves.

PREBIOTICS

Prebiotics are a form of indigestible fibre. They pass through the small intestine and end up in the large intestine, where they provide a feast for waiting microbes. Think of them like fertilizer – they allow your friendly bacteria to grow and multiply.

Breast milk is the first prebiotic we come across. Then, as our diet changes, they come from fibrous foods, the top sources being bananas, asparagus, chicory, Jerusalem artichokes, dandelion leaves, onions, leeks, garlic and raw wheat bran (although other fruit and vegetables, pulses, nuts and seeds contain some prebiotic fibre, as well).

A prebiotic diet has been shown to increase bacteria numbers in the gut, so we can call these sorts of foods 'functional'. It's recommended we have at least 5g (⅛oz) of prebiotic fibre a day, which would be hard to get from one source. So the more and wider variety of vegetables and fruit you can eat each day, the better.

What you do when you're not exercising also counts. Being sedentary all day – which can be hard to avoid if you have a desk-bound or driving job – has been described as a health threat equal to smoking. So we need to move more on a daily, in fact hourly, basis. Just don't go to extremes. Excessive, high-intensity exercise, for too long or too frequently, can also be a stress on the body and mind. It's all about balance.

ANTIBIOTICS

Sometimes antibiotics are still vital to treat infections. We're not suggesting for a moment that you refuse them when needed. But if your illness could be a virus, you'll be better off without.

Another way to avoid antibiotics is to bolster your immunity so you're less likely to become ill. And following a gut-healthy diet like the G Plan is a huge leap in that direction. If you do need a course of antibiotics? Pay extra attention to your diet and consider a probiotic supplement during and after, to help repopulate your gut (*see* page 24).

PROBIOTICS

These are foods that contain live bacteria and yeasts – some are naturally fermented, some have cultures added. The idea is they make it through the digestive tract to the large intestine and help to increase the population and activity of the microbiome.

You've probably heard of probiotics in yogurt and milky drinks that are marketed specifically as functional foods, able to restore your 'natural balance'. Some of these little pots, however, contain added sugar, which can unbalance the microbiome – so they're not actually the best choice.

There's also a vast array of probiotic supplements available in pill or powder form and they can do some good (see page 24). Knowing which strains of bacteria they contain (versus which you need), in what amounts and if they can survive the journey to your gut, however, is another matter.

For now, taking probiotic drinks or supplements can't hurt, but there is only really evidence that they're useful during or after a course of antibiotics or a tummy bug, and for those people suffering with IBS or lactose intolerance.[5]

The best way to benefit then, is to add naturally probiotic fermented foods to your diet (see page 18). And, you guessed it, to include as wide a variety as possible. Choose from kefir, kombucha, kimchi, sauerkraut and other pickles, miso, aged cheese, unsweetened natural 'live' or 'bio' yogurt. They're all acquired tastes but the G Plan helps you to introduce them gradually and reap the benefits.

VARIETY

The Western diet, based as it often is around processed, convenience food and drinks, tends to be limited. Surveys have shown that many of us eat as few as six or seven meals on rotation.[6] The majority of us fail to get our five-a-day of fruit and vegetables[7] and that's a recommended minimum. Many experts suggest it should be seven and some other countries put it as high as nine.

Such limited diets are easy to fall into. Life is very busy, you don't have time or money to shop at markets and green-grocers (if you can find them),

the kids/your partner/flatmates are fussy eaters, you don't want to spend all evening in the kitchen so ready meals and takeaways rule... The advent of seemingly helpful tools like online supermarket shopping only serves to make our diet more samey – you don't shop according to what's in season or what you fancy, but what's on your 'previous orders' list. We understand (and we've been there).

But research shows dieters who eat a greater variety of healthy foods are more likely to lose weight and fat in the long term[8] and less likely to develop metabolic syndrome[9] (associated with type 2 diabetes and heart disease).

Breaking free from the monotony of the 'same old, same old' diet is therefore the fundamental principle of the G Plan. Diversity is your mantra. Write it on some Post-it notes, stick them to your refrigerator, your cupboards or your laptop for next time you do that online order. If you can embrace variety in your diet, your health can't fail to benefit. Choose a rainbow of fruit and vegetables, try new types, eat seasonally, cook new recipes with new ingredients. Get out of that food rut.

It's that simple, and that's what we're going to do. The beauty of the G Plan is that it's not a diet of restriction, rules and taking away. It's about abundance. We want you to branch out, broaden your horizons, enjoy new foods and flavours and a more exciting, varied, natural diet. You'll be surprised how quickly the positive effects appear.

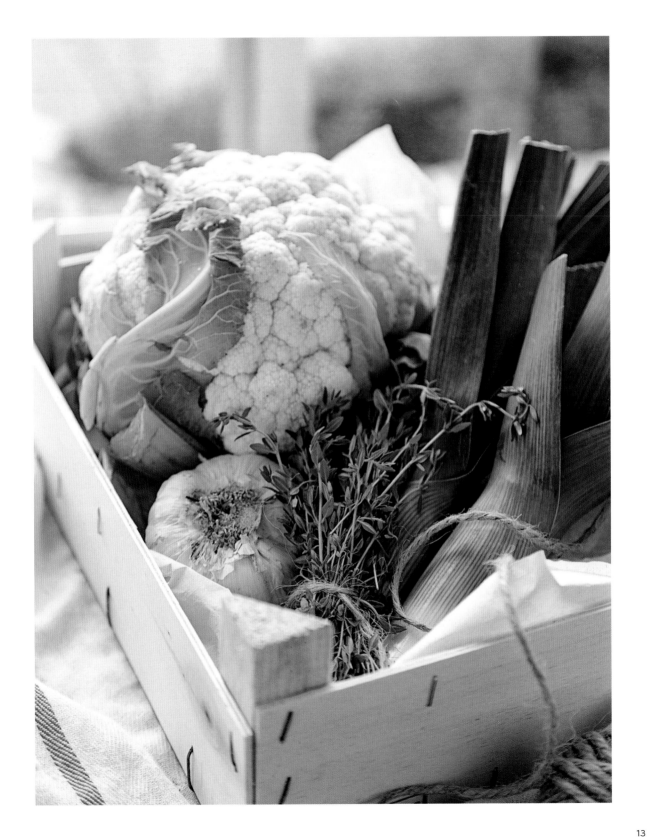

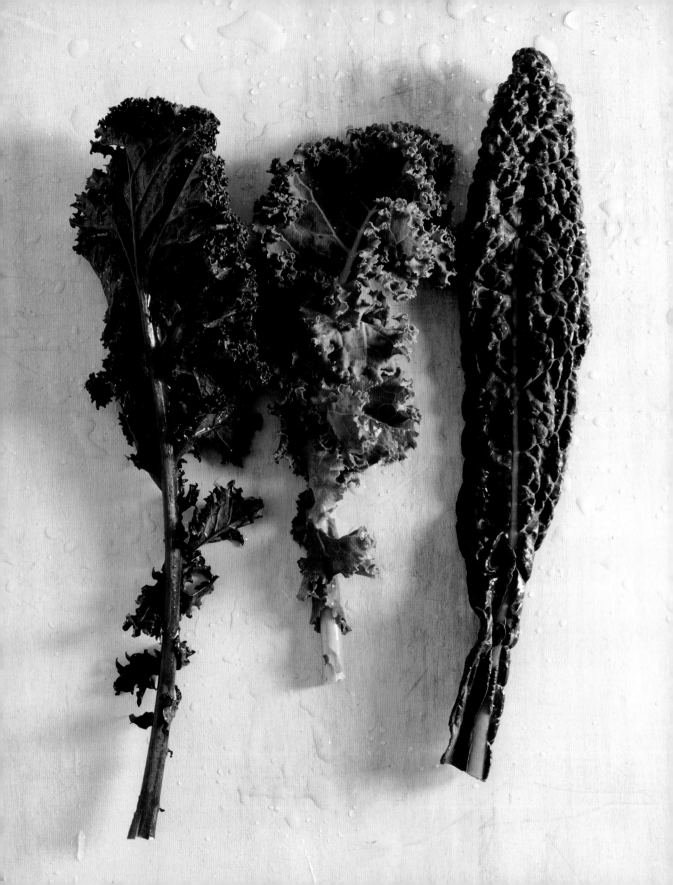

WOULD YOU BENEFIT FROM THE G PLAN DIET?

The short answer is yes. We truly believe that this plan, which works to rest, repair and nourish the gut, is suitable for everyone. It's safe, straightforward, balanced and fad free. Over the 21 days you will move towards a new way of eating, which is focused on diversity and can be maintained for life. You may be particularly keen to try it if you tick any (or all) of the following boxes:

☐ I'd like to lose weight
☐ Other diets don't seem to be working for me
☐ I often feel bloated
☐ I'm lacking in energy
☐ I don't sleep well/I sleep too much
☐ I sometimes experience 'brain fog' and can't think straight
☐ My complexion is congested and spotty
☐ I have other skin issues, like eczema or psoriasis
☐ I suffer from low mood/mood swings
☐ I frequently have a cold/flu/tummy bug
☐ I have PMS/menopausal symptoms
☐ I have recurrent thrush (candida)
☐ I often experience indigestion or heartburn
☐ My digestion is sluggish
☐ I suffer from excess wind
☐ I often experience diarrhoea (perhaps alternating with constipation) and cramps
☐ I have irritable bowel syndrome (IBS)
☐ I have an inflammatory bowel disease (Crohn's, colitis)
☐ Certain foods seem to irritate me
☐ My diet is high in processed foods
☐ I crave/rely too much on sugar/alcohol/caffeine
☐ I rarely cook from scratch
☐ My supermarket shop is always the same
☐ I have the same breakfast every day
☐ I end up eating the same old lunches/dinners most weeks
☐ I've taken lots of antibiotics in the past/I'm on long-term antibiotics

We can't promise that the G Plan will cure all these issues. But we are sure that if you follow the 21-day menu and continue with the new way of eating, you'll be giving your gut – and all the other functions it influences – the best foundation for good health.

We're confident that by allowing your microbiome to flourish, you'll see many of the following benefits:

• Loss of excess weight, usually around 0.5–1kg (1–2lb) a week
• Reduction in water retention
• Reduction in bloating, distension and gas
• Improved energy and alertness
• Better sleep
• Clearer skin
• Improved mood
• Boosted immunity
• Reduced PMS or menopausal symptoms
• Fewer candida episodes
• Improved digestion and elimination
• Some relief from IBS/IBD symptoms
• Increased awareness of true food intolerances
• Fewer cravings
• Renewed interest in shopping for food and cooking with a greater variety of ingredients

Many of these benefits will be tangible within days and will really help to spur you on. Are you ready to make the change and give your gut some TLC? Read on and join the G Plan revolution.

GETTING STARTED ON THE G PLAN

So you're ready. Here's what you can expect for the next 21 days.

The G Plan is designed around three phases: Rest, Re-wild and Rebalance. These will take you to a new and diverse diet, with all the health and weight loss benefits that brings. You'll follow daily menu plans and easy recipes to feel full, alert and energized throughout.

The phased method is something Amanda uses as part of her highly successful nutrition clinics and retreat programmes, as it's an effective way to make lasting changes. This is the new normal.

If weight loss is your goal, before you start, note your weight and key measurements (waist, hips, arms, thighs) and take photographs of yourself in your underwear or workout gear, from the side, front and back. It's also a good idea to keep a food, symptoms and mood diary, which is a simple but effective way to spot possible reactions to foods, as well as monitor factors like your energy levels, skin, mood and weight. It'll keep you motivated as you see how far you've come, and if you find your good habits slipping in the future.

The phases
PHASE 1: REST (5 DAYS)

During this phase, your digestive system will have some well-earned downtime. It's similar to a 'detox' but, as your body detoxifies itself all the time, it is about supporting and optimizing those natural processes. Also, temporarily eliminating common gut irritants and keeping food simple and easy to digest, allows any past tummy troubles to settle.

It also gives your weight loss a kick-start, which is always good motivation. Bloating and water retention will disappear so you'll look and feel lighter in days.

Each day starts with a smoothie, and lunch and dinner are lightly cooked rather than raw. Meals are based around plant foods, wheat-free grains and protein to keep you fuller for longer.

Processed foods, added sugar, alcohol, gluten, dairy, carbonated beverages (even water) and vegetables from the nightshade family (potatoes, tomatoes, aubergines, peppers, etc.) are off limits just for now as they're common irritants.

You'll be limiting your grains (only gluten-free oats and quinoa), keeping caffeine down to a maximum of two cups of green tea a day, and having limited beans and pulses. The foods you eat are all gut soothers, known for their calming, healing effects.

PHASE 2: RE-WILD (9 DAYS)

This is when we start to bring the diversity into your diet that your microbiome loves. We continue with the gut soothers but add in gut boosters, as prebiotics and probiotics. Expect lots of prebiotic vegetables to give your gut flora the nutrients it needs to thrive and proliferate. And we're adding fermented, probiotic foods and drinks according to your tastes and what's on offer where you live. You'll pick from ingredients like kefir, kombucha, pickles and more, to increase microbes in the gut. During these nine days you have a few more breakfast and snack options from which to choose. You're also gradually consuming more beans and pulses and re-introducing eggs.

PHASE 3: REBALANCE (7 DAYS)

By now you'll be feeling great and as if you've really got to grips with this new way of eating. Hopefully you've discovered some new tastes and have a good recipe repertoire, too. This final, seven-day phase is about keeping up the good work and re-introducing the food types we cut out in Phase 1, to see how your digestive system reacts. You can now have a small glass of red wine every few days, if you like (although we recommend other alcohol is kept out of the diet until after the 21 days). Day by day we'll introduce those possible irritants we eliminated in Phase 1, so you can easily tell if you react to them.

Moving forwards

Once you've completed 21 days, it's the beginning of your new way of eating, for life. You've given your digestion a good rest from common irritants and anti-nutrients so your taste buds will have changed and you no longer crave them. After a period of abstinence, foods that used to taste good tend to taste extreme. So you'll find it easy to carry on without those sugary, processed foods, or at least to have them in far smaller amounts. The benefits, including weight loss, can continue as long as you stick within the principles of the G Plan. And it'll feel so easy.

Weigh, measure and photograph yourself again so you can see how far you've come (and do it at regular intervals). Then go to the Moving Forwards section (see page 124), which is full of inspiration for continuing a G Plan way of eating for life.

When should I start?

The G Plan is designed to work in your normal life so you'll be eating enough to keep you firing on all cylinders. That said, a non-working day, when life tends to be easier to manage, might be the best time to start. Don't pile on unnecessary pressure: if you're going through a particularly busy period at work or have lots of social engagements, perhaps wait before embarking on the plan.

Get ready

Planning and preparation are key. All the kitchen gadgets you'll need are a blender or food processor. You'll be doing lots of cooking from scratch, which may feel time consuming at first if you're not used to it, but we've included plenty of recipes for batch-cooking: dinner one evening becomes the next day's lunch or a couple of freezer meals for future use. Stock up on BPA-free plastic containers for freezer storage and packed lunches.

Use the shopping lists provided to make sure you have all the food you'll need. It might feel like you're buying a lot, but think of it like a kitchen makeover. The storecupboard ingredients you have to buy will become new staples, and what you're spending on fresh produce you're saving on processed foods.

If you worry you'll be tempted by foods that are 'off plan', like biscuits or crisps, don't have them in the house. Give them away to a food bank or friend. If family members aren't doing the G Plan and want to continue having them, keep them in a cupboard you don't look in. Out of sight, out of mind.

Make it work for you

This plan is designed to be flexible and adaptable. If you can't get or don't like an ingredient, it's fine to leave it out or substitute something similar (don't like tomatoes? Use red peppers. No almonds? Another nut will do). And the portions are just a guideline. Obviously if weight loss is your focus you won't want to overdo it – and we've deliberately made portions generous. But if you need more – or less – that's fine. If you have vegetables or salad that need using up but they're not in the recipe, don't waste them, throw them in!

What we suggest is that you try to keep to three meals a day. If you want a snack we have suggestions in each phase, but don't have more than two a day (and don't feel you *have* to have them). We want to move away from that idea of grazing throughout the day and get back in touch with hunger cues. That's how our guts function best, too.

Feel energized, keep active

We all know that keeping active is essential for good health – and the microbiome – but it's also important to nurture yourself. Try to follow some of the lifestyle advice we include in each phase, which will be helpful for stress relief and self-care. The first few days of the plan you may be adjusting to the new diet so don't take too much on; stick to exercise you're used to. A good diet supports energy and performance in the long term anyway. This is not the time to take up a new sport, push yourself to the limit at a HIIT (high-intensity interval training) class or sign up for an Ironman. As Hannah found, attempting a hilly, off-road half-marathon, in soaring heat on day 3, is tough! So, go for walks, do some yoga or Pilates, have a gentle run or cycle. Feel free to increase your exercise after the first few days.

TOP 10 GUT-FRIENDLY FOODS

This list is by no means exhaustive and, as you know by now, diversity is the name of the good-gut game. But here's our selection of foods that deserve to be favourites.

1 GARLIC

Garlic is a valuable antioxidant and prebiotic, which provides nutrients including vitamins B6 and C, manganese and selenium. It also contains a compound called allicin, linked with good circulation and heart health, as well as reducing colds and boosting immunity. All that *and* it wards off vampires...

It crops up regularly, raw and cooked, throughout the G Plan, thanks to the flavour it provides alongside health benefits. Part of the same family, onions and leeks are also valuable prebiotic foods, especially when raw.

2 BANANAS

Poor bananas. Their cards are marked by so many diets and so-called healthy eating plans but not this one. We know what prebiotic-packed powerhouses they are. These fibre-rich fruits also top up your potassium levels, making them the perfect pre- or post-exercise snack. We recommend starting your day with a banana-based smoothie to give the good bacteria in your gut a hearty breakfast, too. Convenient and nutritious, it would be rude to say no. Watermelon, grapefruit, peaches and nectarines, dates and figs are also rich in prebiotic fibre.

3 ASPARAGUS

Another prebiotic fibre provider, these delicious spears deserve a regular place in our diets. They're also rich in the B vitamin folate, antioxidant vitamins A, C and E, vitamin K and chromium, and they have diuretic properties to help with water retention. Enjoy it very lightly steamed, grilled or stir-fried. Or, to retain more of the fibre and prebiotic qualities, try it raw. It's surprisingly edible 'shaved' into salads or whizzed into green smoothies.

4 NATURAL YOGURT

This is the best-known gut-friendly food, naturally teeming with probiotic 'live' bacteria, such as lactic acid bacteria (particularly *Lactobacillus acidophilus*) which can pass through the digestive system to the large intestine where it's needed. It's thought that eating probiotics like yogurt can change the microbiome in subtle ways – not just boosting bacteria numbers but improving the function and interactions of what's already there.

Go for a full-fat (organic if possible) live or 'bio' yogurt that's unsweetened. Avoid low-fat or flavoured varieties as these will contain added sugar. Check the ingredients list – it should only contain pasteurized milk and live and active bacterial cultures.

5 FERMENTED VEGETABLES

Also known as pickles, these are an acquired taste but they are worth getting used to – and thanks to the health benefits they're becoming really trendy now. Fermentation is a natural process. But when we talk about fermented vegetables, we mean the type of fermentation that humans have been doing for thousands of years, both to preserve food and add distinct, strong flavours. There are many different ways to ferment food but the basic method (lacto-fermentation) involves soaking vegetables in their own juice, or brine, and allowing bacteria to grow. Sometimes bacterial, fungal or yeast cultures are added, too. The bacteria breaks down all the vegetable sugars and produces lactic acid with a tangy, vinegary taste. It's a flavour that can take some getting used to, but many people love it.

When we eat fermented vegetables (or pickles), we're not only ingesting all that fibre, good bacteria and other nutrients, we're also consuming foods that have already started to break down – so they're easy on the digestion, too.

Sauerkraut is pickled cabbage, available relatively cheaply in the international aisle of most supermarkets. It's a traditional German and Polish staple. Kimchi is a traditional Asian pickle and one many Koreans credit for their longevity. It's usually made from cabbage with added spices, and is available from Asian supermarkets or larger supermarkets.

Keep in mind, though, that not all fermented foods are pickled and not all pickles are fermented. Pickled beetroot, gherkins, onions and the like are preserved in an acidic vinegar. So, even though vinegar is a product of fermentation, the vegetables are not fermented and therefore they don't bring the same benefits.

Try adding sauerkraut, kimchi or other vegetables to a casserole, having them as a side dish or as a topping on soup, rye bread or oatcakes.

6 JERUSALEM ARTICHOKES

Not to be confused with pretty globe artichokes which make great antipasti, Jerusalem artichokes look like knobbly ginger roots and their use is similar to that of potatoes. They taste delicious and work well in soups, roasted or mashed as a side dish, in casseroles and even thinly sliced and made into crisps. One of the top prebiotic vegetables,

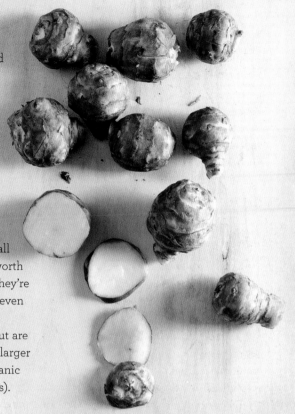

they're also a good source of potassium and iron and have a lower glycaemic index (GI) than potatoes, so will fill you up for longer.

We admit there's that well-known side effect that has led to the nickname 'fartichokes' and they may cause bloating in some people. But in small quantities they're well worth adding to your menu. They're not always easy to find, even when they're in season (November to March) but are worth tracking down in larger supermarkets (or in organic vegetable delivery boxes).

7 KEFIR

First, let's get the pronunciation right: it's 'kee-fer' (as in Sutherland). Next, let's get on board with the belly benefits. Kefir is basically like a live yogurt drink, but with as much as three times the probiotic power. It originated in Eastern Europe and the name comes from the Turkish word *keif* (as in Richards), meaning 'good feeling'. It's made by adding kefir 'grains' to any dairy or plant/nut milk. The grains provide a live colony of bacteria and yeast which all ferment with the milk, producing lots of bacteria species known to benefit our microbiome. You'll find plenty of uses for it as you work through the G Plan. And in addition to the bacteria, you'll

benefit from many other nutrients: protein, calcium, potassium, folic acid, lactic acid, biotin, vitamins K and B.

These days kefir can be found fairly cheaply at most supermarkets (located in the chilled, Polish section). It can be made with plant and nut milks (such as coconut), as well as dairy. The bottle is normally white and shouldn't say anything other than 'kefir' or 'natural kefir'. You can also find it in health-food shops, with different flavours, but these can be a bit pricier. On the ingredients list you just want pasteurized milk and live kefir/ bacterial cultures – and sometimes kefir yeast. Make sure there are no added sugars.

8 NUTS AND SEEDS

These are another food staple that are often on the 'banned' list in weight-loss diets, because they're relatively high in calories. But they're an amazing source of unsaturated essential fats, protein, fibre and minerals, as well as being prebiotics and known to enhance the diversity of the microbiome.

Studies suggest our microbes feed off the fatty acids and polyphenols in nuts (and those in olive oil), breaking them down into smaller compounds which help to lower lipid levels and boost the immune system. Polyphenols help the microbiome to diversify and flourish, and prevent unwanted microbes that might cause infection. Other studies have shown nuts can suppress appetite and promote weight loss.[10] So we're putting nuts and seeds right back on the YES list.

Go for as wide a variety as possible and choose unroasted and unsalted nuts and seeds – you can always toast and season them yourself with spices (*see* page 114). They are moreish but they're also filling, so eat slowly and enjoy in moderation – one snack should be around 30g (1oz).

9 MISO

Miso is a Japanese seasoning made from fermenting soya beans, barley and brown rice, so it gets another cheer from your large intestine, which loves the probiotics it provides. It has that delicious, savoury umami taste. You can buy it as a paste from larger and Asian supermarkets and use it to make savoury dips and dressings, or add to soups, stocks and casseroles (at the end of cooking, to preserve the probiotics). Or simply stir a spoonful into hot water to make your own miso soup, which is really tasty and filling. Keep some sachets in your bag or your desk drawer at work and you have a healthy snack in seconds. It's also available from many high-street café chains now, too.

10 KOMBUCHA

Another ancient elixir that has recently been appropriated by savvy hipsters, kombucha is a fermented tea drink. It has a slight fizz and clean, vinegary taste – we're not really selling it to you here, are we? But honestly, once you get used to it, it's a palatable, tangy tonic, so teeming with probiotics you feel instantly virtuous on imbibing it.

Historically, it was brewed at home using a mixture of black or green tea and sugar, with a starter culture called a SCOBY (symbiotic colony of bacteria and yeast). This flat, beige disc helps to ferment the ingredients and the result is an acidic 'functional beverage' that has also been found to contain enzymes, polyphenols, amino acids, B vitamins and vitamin C. If you fancy having a go at brewing your own, see our guide opposite. Otherwise, various ready-brewed drinks are commercially available – your best bet is a health-food shop chiller cabinet or buying online. Many are flavoured to make them less tart, but do check for added sugar and avoid the products that contain it.

Ready-brewed kombucha can be expensive though, and it's relatively easy to make your own once you've acquired a SCOBY and 'starter liquid', either from another brewer or from an online kombucha starter kit. Keep all equipment, surfaces and your hands clean to avoid contamination.

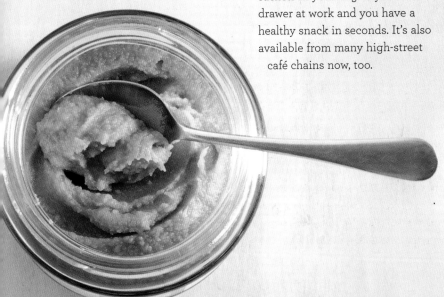

BREWING YOUR OWN KOMBUCHA

First, sterilize your jar. Preheat the oven to 140°C (275°F) Gas Mark 1. Wash the jar in warm, soapy water and rinse well. Place the wet jar upside down on a baking tray and put in the oven for 15 minutes, until dry.

Infuse the tea with 400ml (14fl oz) boiling water for 10–15 minutes.

Strain the tea into a measuring jug, add the sugar and stir through until dissolved.

Pour into the sterilized pickling jar and top up with 2 litres (3½ pints) of cold water. Allow to cool to room temperature.

Stir the starter kombucha into the tea mixture and put the SCOBY on top. The kombucha increases the acidity of the liquid to speed up the fermentation process.

Cover the jar with a cloth and secure with the elastic band. This will protect it from dust and flies while still allowing air in.

Transfer to a warm (20–29°C/68–85°F) dark place where the jar won't be knocked or disturbed.

Leave for 7–10 days. The mixture will become 'fizzy' as the bacteria and yeast in SCOBY feed off the sugar.

The longer you leave it, the more acidic it will become, so you may like to try it earlier to suit your taste. Remove the cloth and push the SCOBY to one side to take a teaspoonful to try.

If you have a pH meter or test strips (available cheaply online) you can test the acidity of your kombucha. Ideally it should be between 2.5 and 3.5. Or you can just taste it. It should be not too sweet, not too vinegary.

When it has reached your desired taste, your kombucha is finished. Carefully take out the SCOBY (store this in a small clip-lock jar along with 200ml/7fl oz of the kombucha liquid for your next batch, which you can start straightaway).

Transfer the rest of the kombucha to bottles – ideally swing-top bottles with a lid that can withstand some pressure – and store in the refrigerator. Like wine, many people say kombucha improves with age.

If you like, you can make a 'second fermentation' at this stage. Simply add a little fruit to each bottle. This will ferment and increase the fizziness of each drink as well as adding flavour. Open and close the caps each night to release some of the pressure and taste them after 3–5 days.

MAKES ABOUT 2 LITRES (3½ PINTS)

EQUIPMENT

large glass pickling jar (at least 2 litres/3½ pints)
a teapot or saucepan
large 2-litre (3½-pint) measuring jug
clean square of muslin/cloth
large elastic band
pH meter or pH test strips (optional)
small clip-lock jar
large swing top glass bottles, for storage

INGREDIENTS

3–4 black or green tea bags (or 3–4 teaspoons of leaves in a metal infuser ball)
160g (5¾oz) granulated white sugar
about 200ml (7fl oz) 'starter' kombucha (saved from your last batch or supplied with your SCOBY)
a SCOBY (symbiotic colony of bacteria and yeast)

AND THE GUT FOES

There are very few foods that are off limits on the G Plan because your diet should be as broad as possible. But there are some key groups that are anti-nutrients for your gut. They should be eliminated for the 21 day-plan and then kept to a minimum moving forwards. Once you have completed the 21 days you'll most likely find that you didn't miss them and no longer need them.

SUGAR

Links to obesity and diabetes aside, all sugars (check labels for anything ending in '-ose', particularly high-fructose corn syrup) are bad news for your microbiome. It feeds pathogenic organisms such as *Candida*, which can then suppress growth of friendly bacteria. Sugar, refined carbohydrates and processed foods are also absorbed more quickly in the small intestine, leaving gut microbes hungry. The theory goes they then 'snack' on your gut lining, causing leaky gut.

REFINED STARCHY CARBOHYDRATES

The process to make 'white' versions of food staples like flour, bread, rice and pasta means much of the fibre and other nutrients have been removed. They raise blood sugar levels faster and won't fill you up for as long. Once digested, they behave like sugar, reducing gut flora. Some people with IBS will find wholegrain 'brown' varieties harder to digest (try them in small amounts) but in general they're the better choice.

ARTIFICIAL SWEETENERS

Not the magic bullet for obesity that they first appeared to be, artificial sweeteners in drinks have been associated with weight gain and diabetes.[11] It's thought they alter appetite and reward pathways in the brain, and lead to increased insulin resistance.[12] Animal studies have shown they reach the large intestine and interact with gut microbes, reducing count and diversity.[13]

ADDITIVES AND PRESERVATIVES

Preservatives are often added to foods and drinks containing artificial sweeteners, because they lack the natural preservation sugar gives. Check labels for chemicals like nitrites and nitrates, MSG, tartrazine, benzoates and citric or phosphorus acid. Along with other additives like colorants, they're likely to have a similar effect on our microbes, reducing their number and diversity. They may also affect immunity, and have been linked with allergies.[14]

PROCESSED FOODS

Most processed foods contain added sugar or sweeteners, often excess salt and saturated fat, and usually additives and preservatives. The best way to know what's in your food, and the effect it might have on your gut and overall health, is to choose natural foods and cook from scratch.

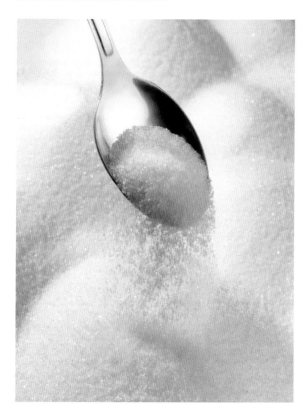

Common Gut Irritants

It's also a good idea not to have too much of these:

ALCOHOL

A depressant and high in sugar, excess alcohol can cause weight gain, has a negative effect on the microbiome and may contribute to leaky gut. Excess consumption also has links to heart and liver disease and some cancers. It's acceptable from Phase 3 onwards, but in small amounts.

GLUTEN

Gluten-containing grains are so prevalent in Western diets that we could all do with cutting down. Much of the benefit of removing gluten is that you are forced to make better choices overall, which means fewer grab-and-go beige foods. You may well find that without gluten you feel better as a whole.

When you reintroduce gluten in the final phase, how you feel will determine whether you should continue to avoid it or just cut down. If you have a gluten intolerance or coeliac disease, clearly gluten should not be reintroduced.

MEAT

While it is beneficial for most people to include meat in their diet a few times a month for the nutrients it provides, much of the meat we eat contains low-level antibiotics which disrupt gut flora. Choose organic if you can or select meat that's been reared in a more natural way.

SATURATED FAT

An animal study conducted in Sweden found that the type of fat we eat is really important for shaping microbial communities and their function.[15] A diet high in saturated animal fats had a negative effect on gut diversity, while one higher in essential fatty acids (fish oils) was beneficial.

It's quite easy to achieve a good fat balance, simply by avoiding the processed foods that saturates are commonly found in. Quit the pies, pastries, cakes, biscuits, fast food and takeaways and you've probably eliminated the majority from your diet. A small

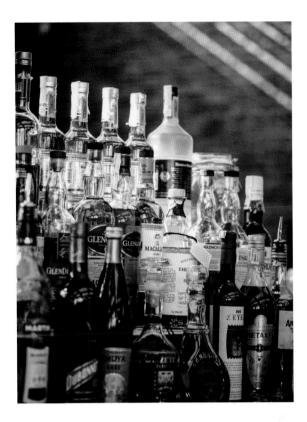

amount from good-quality meat and dairy is fine. Dairy produce, if you can tolerate it, provides valuable vitamins and minerals and has a positive effect on the microbiome. Indeed butter and cheese consumption is linked with an increase in butyrate, a compound produced by microbes that's linked with reduced cholesterol, increased energy and plays a role in fighting obesity.[16]

Coconut oil and milk – which you'll find in some of our recipes – may also be beneficial. The saturated fats in coconut oil are medium-chain triglycerides. They're more rapidly used by the body as fuel and less likely to be stored as fat. So they may have a small metabolism-boosting effect. Just keep in mind that all fats are energy dense, so don't go overboard if you want to keep weight in check.

SUPPLEMENTS

When you're on a health kick, it's tempting to go into a health-food shop or supermarket and stock up on pills, powders, tinctures and elixirs, all promising increased vitality. While we are in favour of many such health products, there are a few caveats well worth mentioning.

First, diet and lifestyle changes should always be a priority. No supplement will magically give positive health effects while you're still following a limited, unbalanced diet. Save your money until you know you're eating and living better. In theory, if you have a diverse, well-balanced diet, such as the G Plan, you shouldn't need too much extra help.

Second, while many products have useful therapeutic benefits, as discussed below, there's no point trying them all at once. If you want to relieve constipation, say, and you try three approaches, how will you know which has worked? Introduce them one or two at a time – more isn't always better.

Third, if you prefer not to take or can't afford any supplements, don't worry. As the name suggests, they're optional extras.

Should I take probiotics?

From yogurts with miracle claims and milky drink 'shots', to all manner of pills and powders, you'd be forgiven for feeling confused about probiotics. Should you take a daily probiotic supplement?

Again, the clue's in the name with supplements. They're an adjunct to a healthy diet, not a panacea. So yes, supporting your health by taking a probiotic is unlikely to harm and may very well do some good. But it's not absolutely necessary – and good food comes first.

What probiotics do is deliver a dose of beneficial bacteria down to your gut. Most products will contain *Lactobacillus* and *Bifidobacterium* strains. Overall these support your beneficial flora. The trouble is that everyone's microbiome is unique and science can't yet identify which strains of bacteria *you* most need, or know which strains are likely to interact to achieve certain benefits. Currently, there haven't been enough large, long-term studies into the benefits of taking probiotics. So scientists can't promise that taking a probiotic will have any specific effects, although the general consensus is that they are helpful overall.

This is all changing fast though. We're starting to understand more about why probiotics work and what they do in the gut. And in the not-too-distant future, this will mean scientists can use them to target specific health conditions and diseases. Experts believe within the next five to ten years, we could be taking probiotics as we do over-the-counter pharmaceutical drugs.

We do know that if you have taken a course of antibiotics, your gut flora will be much depleted by them – collateral damage if you like – and the balance of the microbiome alters. This can lead to less friendly bacteria taking over. Yeast infections (with *Candida albicans)* can take hold and suppress good bacteria further. In severe cases, the pathogenic bacteria *Clostridium difficile* (also known as *C. diff*) can run rampage – it's common in elderly, hospitalized people.

What's also known is that probiotics can help prevent this. Clinical trials have shown that giving hospital patients on antibiotics a three-week course of probiotics significantly reduces the risk of a *C. diff* infection.[17] So if you're taking a course of antibiotics, there's good evidence that taking probiotics during and afterwards can help to restore your microbiome. Equally, if you've had a tummy bug or are experiencing particular digestive issues, probiotics are likely to help.

Quality counts so choose a trusted brand with the maximum potency and diversity of bacteria on the ingredients list. Find the product with the most bacteria per capsule. Steer clear of the yogurts and milk drinks (apart from natural products and kefir) – they tend to be loaded with sugar which simply negates the benefits. Children need slightly different strains so if you're buying for them, choose a product designed for kids – you can get powders that are easy to stir into milk, porridge or yogurt.

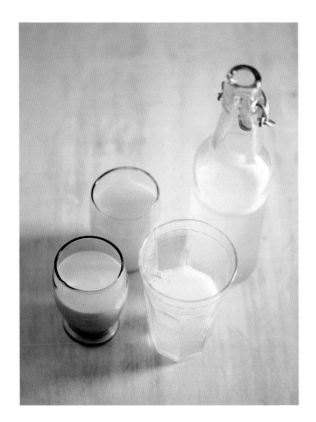

Gut-friendly nutrients

The following nutrients will all be delivered by a diet like the G Plan. However, as they all have specific roles in digestive health and/or weight loss, some people may like to take a supplement. Follow the packet instructions as each supplement will differ.

MAGNESIUM

This mineral is important for gut tone and peristalsis, the function that moves food through the intestines. Known for relieving muscle cramps, it may be useful for those who suffer IBS and/or period pain. It also helps turn the food you eat into energy. If your diet is rich in green leafy vegetables, nuts and brown rice, with some fish, meat and dairy, you should get plenty of magnesium. However, a supplement may be of some help for people with constipation, as may a potassium supplement, although a diet such as the G Plan also provides this. If you don't want to pop a pill, the latest products deliver the mineral through the skin, in the form of bath salts, oil sprays and creams.

B VITAMINS

Vital for mood and energy, this set of vitamins is found in proteins, such as fish, poultry, meat and dairy, as well as green leafy vegetables and pulses. They help with the formation of red blood cells, and process and release energy from your food. Although they each have distinct roles, the various B vitamins work best in synergy, so look for a 'B Complex' formulation, rather than individual supplements.

VITAMIN C

This vitamin, abundant in berries, citrus fruits, tomatoes, peppers and broccoli, is an antioxidant which fights free-radical damage and bolsters immunity. It's also vital for digestion as it supports healthy teeth and gums and helps your body absorb iron. All the connective tissues in your digestive tract contain collagen and vitamin C is vital for its production in the body (and as a bonus, your skin will look younger, too). A regular intake helps to keep the digestive tract strong and repair any damage to its lining. If you choose to supplement, don't take too much as it can cause diarrhoea.

VITAMIN D

Many people are deficient in vitamin D without knowing it. Although you can get small amounts in food (some fish, liver, egg yolks, fortified bread and cereal), the vast majority is synthesized in the body on exposure to sunlight. This means that northern Europeans, who see less sunlight overall, are more vulnerable to a deficiency. Anyone who regularly (and sensibly) uses sunscreen, covers most of their body with clothing, or spends a lot of time indoors, as well as pregnant women, should take a supplement and may even be prescribed one by their doctor.

Vitamin D plays a key role in nerve, immune system and muscle function, as well as helping your body absorb calcium, needed for healthy bones and teeth. A recent study associated healthy vitamin D levels with a reduced risk of colorectal cancers.[18] And another found low levels (and a need for supplements) in people with inflammatory bowel disease (IBD), such as Crohn's and colitis.[19]

We recommend everyone takes a daily supplement, at least through the autumn and winter. The rest of the year, try to let your face and arms see the sun, without protection but before burning, for around 30 minutes a day.

ESSENTIAL FATS

In a varied diet, all fats have a role to play and saturated fats like butter, cheese and full-fat yogurt can contribute to good gut health in moderation. Monounsaturated fatty acids (MUFAs) – plant-based fats found in avocados, nuts and seeds, olives, plant oils and even dark chocolate – are beneficial, too.

However, the only type of fat of which we would benefit from supplmenting is the polyunsaturated fatty acid (PUFA) omega-3. Omega-3s have an anti-inflammatory action in the body, which is useful for all aspects of health, not least IBD. Recent research, presented in Stockholm in 2014, found the omega-3 oils EPA and DHA, present in fish oils, can reduce inflammation and increase beneficial bacteria to protect against gastrointestinal (GI) complaints.[20]

If you're not vegetarian or vegan, a daily omega-3 essential fatty acid supplement could be beneficial, especially if you find it hard to consume two or more portions of oily fish (salmon, trout, mackerel, sardines, fresh tuna) each week. If you are vegetarian, try an algae supplement.

Gut soothers
PSYLLIUM HUSKS

These are a natural, bulk-forming laxative and can be incredibly helpful if you suffer from constipation or a sluggish bowel. The husks soak up water in your gut and make bowel movements softer and easier. We haven't used them in the G Plan recipes because they swell so much in water it's not practical. Instead, you need to take them separately. Stir a teaspoonful into a glass of water and drink before the mixture becomes too gelatinous. It goes without saying that these alone aren't the solution to constipation – working on the overall health of your microbiome is paramount. Use them when needed, or daily for overall digestive health and regularity.

CHIA SEEDS

Chia also swells in water to form a 'chia pudding' and acts in a similar way to psyllium, although it works better in food so you'll find it in the smoothie and breakfast pot recipes (*see* pages 42–8). Because it can absorb up to 12 times its own weight in water, chia is a good hydrating food and anecdotal claims say it helps boost energy, too. It's a great way to improve hydration before exercise. Chia seeds are also high in fibre, so act as good bowel cleansers.

Gut boosters
SPIRULINA

This is a blue-green algae and one of the oldest life forms on earth. It uses light, warmth, water and minerals to produce protein, carbohydrates, vitamins and other vital nutrients. These are all concentrated into a food source rich in amino acids, beta-carotene and iron, among other nutrients, which is easy to digest. It's no wonder it's often described as a superfood. This powerful antimicrobial is a good supplement for anyone who suffers with candida.[21] This may be because it promotes the growth of healthy bacteria in the gut, which prevents the proliferation of candida. It's also thought to help strengthen immunity. While the taste may take a little getting used to, it's easily hidden in green smoothies and soups.

RAW CACAO

Dark chocolate consumption has long been linked to cardiovascular benefits and improved insulin sensitivity. Experts now think that could be due to the anti-inflammatory compounds produced by gut microbes when they get to grips fermenting cocoa (or cacao, the raw form of the cocoa bean). They also seem to stimulate the production of healthier microbes, leading to greater gut diversity.

Gram for gram, raw cacao has the highest concentration of flavonoids of any food. Flavonoids are the same family of polyphenols as those found in nuts and olives, which have antioxidant, anti-inflammatory and microbial benefits. One clinical trial gave volunteers cocoa-derived flavonoids for

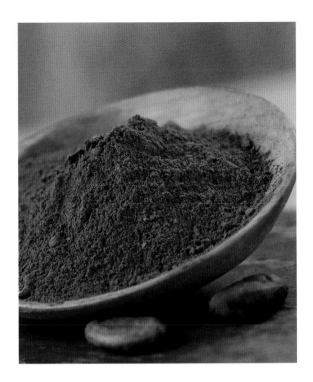

CHICORY ROOT POWDER

Chicory is a woody plant from the dandelion family and you may have enjoyed its leaves (radicchio or endive) in salads. When it comes to gut health, it's the root that is of interest as it contains inulin, a source of soluble fibre and a powerful prebiotic food. It's most readily available as a powdered extract, and available from health-food shops. The flavour is similar to coffee, so it's often found in coffee-substitute products, or you can use it to make your own (*see* page 51). You can also take it on its own as a healthy supplement, or try adding it to smoothies.

L-GLUTAMINE

This is an amino acid, a building block of protein, which is found in animal proteins and some plant foods. A good source is our homemade chicken stock (*see* page 60). L-glutamine stimulates the regeneration of the intestinal mucus which acts as a 'home' and a source of nourishment for bacteria. It is thought it may help to heal ulcers and a leaky gut.[23] This is a condition that occurs when the gut lining becomes abnormally permeable (known as 'intestinal hyperpermeability'), allowing things to pass through to your bloodstream that are normally blocked — like toxins, undigested food particles and other harmful substances. It's been linked to many symptoms, ranging from joint pain and fatigue to allergies, IBD and autoimmune conditions.

L-glutamine may also help to stabilize blood sugar levels and therefore reduce cravings. If you suffer from any of the symptoms or conditions described above, or you have IBS type symptoms, you may benefit from taking a supplement of L-glutamine. It can also be taken as a general gut boost but, again, it's not essential.

four weeks and found significant improvements in their microbiome.[22]

How do you get the benefits? Choose good-quality dark chocolate (not milk chocolate which contains too much fat and sugar) and enjoy a couple of small squares a day once you've completed your 21-day G Plan diet. You can even find bars made with raw cacao in health-food shops these days.

During the diet, you'll find that raw cacao powder or nibs are used in our smoothies and sweet snacks. You can buy both in health-food shops. Always choose raw as the 'normal' cocoa you might use for baking is roasted at high temperatures, destroying many of the nutrients. Raw cacao is cold pressed, better preserving the nutritional value of the cocoa bean. Its living enzymes are preserved but the fat (cacao butter) is removed.

PHASE 1: REST

The first five days of the G Plan are called Rest. They're about giving your digestive system a bit of a break, removing some of the foods that can irritate the gut and getting rid of those that aren't good for the microbiome. You'll still eat well during this phase, you'll feel energized and won't be hungry. But all the meals are light and easy to digest.

Before you get started, make sure you've got everything you need. You'll find a shopping list of ingredients on page 31.

Phase 1 breakfast smoothies

For the next five days, start your day with a mug of hot water flavoured with a slice of lemon and a few thin slices of fresh root ginger if you like. Follow this with any of the smoothie recipes from page 42 onwards. They're all based on bananas, which contain gut-friendly prebiotic fibre. If you're not a fan of banana, adjust the recipes so they include less. You're free to choose whichever smoothie takes your fancy and suits your tastes. But do aim for a different one each day – increasing the variety in your diet starts now. All you need is a blender.

Phase 1 lunches and dinners

To make it as easy as possible to follow this plan, we've created a simple menu with dinners you can reuse for lunch the next day (or vice versa, depending on your schedule). Some of the recipes will also be used in Phases 2 and 3, so where you see this symbol in the recipe section 🍲, be sure to batch-cook and refrigerate or freeze the dish for a quick and simple supper the next day or later on in the plan. The recipes and batch-cooking pointers can be found from page 40.

Phase 1 snacks

If you feel hungry between meals try drinking a glass of water or a herbal tea before reaching for a snack. If you still feel hungry, choose one of the following snack choices, which balance protein and carbs to sustain your energy until your next meal. The recipes can be found from page 110. These snacks can be eaten at any time during the G Plan, but try to limit yourself to two snacks a day.

- **Courgette & Coriander Hummus (see page 116)**
- **Almond Butter or Cashew Nut Dip (see page 115)**
- **Sweet Seeds (see page 114)**
- **Savoury Nuts & Seeds (see page 114)**

Phase 1 drinks

Stick to water and caffeine-free herbal teas in Phase 1. If you find it hard to drink pure water, try adding a few slices of citrus fruit, root ginger, cucumber or mint leaves for subtle but sugar-free flavour. If you usually have caffeine and are worried you'll get withdrawal headaches, you could include green or matcha green tea, just limit yourself to one or two cups per day. Avoid sugary or artificially sweetened diet drinks, ready-made juices and alcohol. Although fresh juices are great for you, we've focused on hassle-free smoothies in the G Plan.

It's a nice ritual to make your own herbal tea infusions, which you can enjoy hot or chilled. Select individual herbs or use several. There's also a huge variety of good-quality ready-made blends available if you don't have the time or ingredients to make your own. Look out for:

- **Chamomile – relaxing, calming and antispasmodic**
- **Lavender – relieves anxiety and aids sleep**
- **Rose – soothing and smells wonderful**
- **Peppermint – helps disperse wind and relieve indigestion**
- **Ginger – eases nausea and calms the gastro-intestinal tract**
- **Fennel – aids digestion and adds sweetness (good after meals if you have a sweet tooth)**

How you might feel during Phase 1

This very much depends on what your diet was like before starting the plan. If it was heavy on processed foods, sugar, bread and caffeine, then the next few days will be quite a change for you. Many people experience withdrawal headaches or fatigue for a couple of days if they go without caffeine. This is thought to be due to temporary changes in brain activity and blood flow to the brain caused by the abstinence.[24] If that's the case for you, one or two cups of green tea in the morning can help to ease the transition, providing just enough caffeine along with a good dose of antioxidant polyphenols. Any headaches should subside after a couple of days.

One of the most positive early changes people report is feeling much less bloated and gassy, with a flatter tummy. This is because we've eliminated those common gut irritants, which you may not even have known caused those symptoms. Water retention often disappears, too, because you will be better hydrated and be eating more vegetables and fewer processed foods high in hidden salt. And seeing and feeling those changes is a great incentive to keep going.

Don't be surprised if your usual bowel habits change over the next few days, too. If you're eating in a different way, your digestion will reflect that. The menu plan features foods that are easy to digest, so it's normal for them to pass through you quite quickly! You're likely to see your regularity improve over the course of the 21 days, as the plant food and fibre in your diet increases.

It's a good idea to keep a track of any physical and emotional changes, using a food, symptoms and mood diary. If you notice any of your digestive issues worsen rather than get better on the plan, or you have any new symptoms, this can help you to identify possible triggers.

Keep active

It should be entirely possible for you to continue with your normal exercise routine on the G Plan. As we've said, this first phase may not be the time to take up a new workout or set yourself a gruelling fitness challenge. But we'd absolutely encourage you to stay fit and active, and you'll be well nourished and energized to do so.

If you don't exercise much at the moment, try to build more activity into your days. Start by making time for a 10-minute brisk walk twice a day, adding five minutes each day until you're walking for 30 minutes at a time. Yoga and Pilates are a good fit, too.

Time for you

Try to make this phase a rest for mind as well as body. If you start at a weekend or quieter time, could you have a break from technology? Get stuck into a novel, enjoy cooking, spend time outdoors in nature.

Before a shower or bath, try dry-skin body brushing, to boost your lymph circulation and drainage. Using a soft-bristled brush, sweep all over your body in the direction of your heart. This is particularly useful if you have a very sedentary job or mobility issues.

Have a relaxing mineral bath with magnesium salts, also known as Epsom salts. Look after your skin with a nourishing body oil or lotion (add a couple of drops of relaxing lavender or detoxifying juniper essential oils to a handful of lotion) and take time for some self-massage.

If you're familiar with meditation, have a short session morning and evening. If you're not, don't be daunted. Something as simple as a breathing exercise can help to calm your mind and focus you for the day ahead – or wind down for the evening.

- **Find somewhere quiet where you can sit or lie down comfortably.**
- **Close your eyes.**
- **Place your hands lightly over your belly.**
- **Become aware of your breathing; don't try to change it, simply be aware of its pattern.**
- **Feel the cool air entering through your nostrils, the warm air leaving. How does it sound? How does it feel?**
- **Gradually move your concentration to your belly – what can you feel under your hands as you breathe? If you're breathing fully and deeply, you should feel your belly rise on your inhalation and fall as you exhale.**
- **Now make your breathing a little deeper. Breathe in for a slow count of four, feeling your belly rise.**
- **Hold for a count of four, making sure that you stay relaxed.**

- Breathe out for a count of four, feeling your belly contract.
- Hold for four.
- Repeat this exercise slowly for a few rounds, then let your breathing return to normal.
- When you're ready, open your eyes.

This exercise can be effective for relieving anxiety or panic and it's something you can do any time, anywhere – even on a packed train during rush hour.

	LUNCH	DINNER
DAY 1	Quinoa Salad with Pesto Dressing & Toasted Seeds (page 63)	Warming Broth with protein of your choice (page 61)
DAY 2	Warming Broth topped with toasted seeds (page 61)	Vegetable & Ginger Casserole with protein of your choice (page 64)
DAY 3	Vegetable & Ginger Casserole with quinoa (page 64)	Creamy Broccoli Pesto Soup (page 67)
DAY 4	Creamy Broccoli Pesto Soup with added greens and crunchy seeds (page 67)	Turmeric Lentil Bake (page 69)
DAY 5	Turmeric Lentil Bake (page 69)	Coconut Carrot Soup (page 70)

PHASE 1 SHOPPING LIST

BREAKFASTS

You won't need to buy everything in the following list – if you choose your five breakfast smoothies for Phase 1 in advance, you only need to buy the ingredients for those.

Fresh ingredients

Avocados
Bananas (enough for one per day)
Blueberries (fresh or frozen)
Coconut water
Fresh mint and ginger
Lemons and limes
Mixed berries (fresh or frozen)
Non-dairy milk
Papaya
Passion fruit
Spinach
Strawberries (fresh or frozen)

Storecupboard ingredients

Almond butter
Cayenne pepper
Chia seeds
Cinnamon
Desiccated coconut
Flaxseeds
Gluten-free oats
Green tea
Silken tofu
Spirulina
Turmeric

LUNCHES, DINNERS AND SNACKS

Fresh ingredients

Avocados
Broccoli
Carrots
Celeriac
Celery
Cucumber
Fresh basil, ginger, coriander, parsley
Garlic
Lemons and limes
Onions and leeks
Pumpkin/butternut squash
Spinach
Swede
Almond milk
Chicken breast and/ or legs
Chicken carcass (if making your own stock)
Salmon
Tempeh
Tofu
White fish

Storecupboard ingredients

Apple cider vinegar (if making your own stock)
Bay leaves
Black pepper
Cashew nuts
Ground spices (Chinese five spice, ground cinnamon, cumin, smoked paprika and tumeric)
Coconut milk
Coconut oil
Dried thyme
Gluten-free oatcakes
Ground almonds
Kaffir lime leaves (optional)
Olive oil (mild and cold-pressed extra virgin)
Quinoa
Red lentils
Sea salt flakes and black pepper
Seeds for toasting (sesame, pumpkin, sunflower or a mix)
Tahini
Tamari soy sauce
Vegetable or chicken stock (if not making your own)
Whole almonds

PHASE 2: RE-WILD

The next days, Re-wild, work on repopulating your gut with the friends it needs. You've given your digestive system a rest and allowed any inflammation to calm down. So now we're bringing in prebiotics and probiotics to nourish, nurture, support and build the beneficial bacteria in your gut.

There's more flexibility in this phase and you have more choice when it comes to breakfasts and snacks. If you find you need to swap days around or adapt recipes to suit eating out, that's fine. You've learned enough to be able to stick within the framework and rules of the G Plan. Embrace the diversity and explore the new foods and flavours Phase 2 brings. You – and your gut – will really enjoy this new phase of eating.

As before, get ready by checking the refrigerator and cupboards to see which items from the Phase 2 Shopping List you'll need to buy (see page 35).

Phase 2 breakfasts

For the nine days of this phase, continue to start your day with hot water, lemon and optional ginger. For breakfast you may still choose any of the smoothies (see page 42). The difference is that you can now add the gut-boosting Phase 2 extras (if you like), or you can try one of the breakfast alternatives below. The recipes for these can be found from page 48. 'Diversity' remains your mantra so try to avoid picking your favourite choice or the easiest option every morning. Can you choose something different each day? Go on... your gut will thank you.

- **Coconut Cinnamon Chia Pot (see page 48)**
- **Mixed Seed Porridge (see page 51)**
- **Healthy Cooked Breakfast (see page 52)**

Phase 2 lunches and dinners

These meals build on the ingredients and recipes used in Phase 1, with some added substance and gut-boosting extras. You should feel as if you're eating more now but it's all still light and easy on the digestion. The recipes for Phase 2 can be found from page 72 onwards.

Phase 2 snacks

Now we've added eggs and kefir into the plan, you can add the following delicious and nutritious options to your snack choices.

- **Hard-boiled eggs**
- **Kefir with nuts and seeds, apple, berries or cinnamon**
- **Chickpea Hummus (see page 116) with vegetable crudités or gluten-free oatcakes**

When selecting your snacks, think about what you're having for breakfast, lunch and dinner that day and try not to double up if there's an alternative that would increase the range of foods in your diet. For example, if you've had kefir for breakfast, go for an egg as a snack and vice versa.

Phase 2 drinks

Continue to stay hydrated with water and herbal or green teas. At this stage, carbonated water is fine, too. Other herbal teas can be introduced, including turmeric, for its anti-inflammatory action, or nettle, a cleansing and energizing herb rich in B vitamins. If you have caffeine (in green tea), stick to one or two cups per day. If you're craving coffee, try one or two cups a day of our prebiotic Caffeine-free Chicory Root 'Coffee' (see page 51). You can also introduce probiotic-packed kombucha (see page 21).

How you might feel during Phase 2

By now, any headaches and lethargy from reducing caffeine and sugar will have subsided. You should be feeling the benefits of being better hydrated – more energy, clearer skin, brighter eyes, no dark circles. Without the ups and downs that sugar and caffeine cause, your moods, energy and focus should feel more even. Sugar cravings? They're history.

If you have very sensitive digestion, there's a chance you might find the introduction of some of the new functional foods causes a reaction. The key is not to avoid them but to reduce the amount you have.

Just add a splash of kefir to your smoothie, for example, gradually increasing the amount. If you have IBS or an IBD, some of the more fibrous vegetables may trigger a flare-up, so eat lightly cooked vegetables rather than raw. Having been through Phase 1 to rest and heal your gut, they're far less likely to be a problem for you now. But stick with your food diary so you can monitor your responses and adjust amounts and recipes accordingly. Ideally, keep in as many of these foods as you can. Don't worry about gurgling digestion, that's quite normal and just your body doing its job!

You're more tuned in to your hunger cues now and, as such, you might find some of the suggested portions too big. They're just a guideline so eat slowly, mindfully, listen to your body and if you're full, stop. If you want more, that's also fine. It's all good.

Keep active

As you're feeling more energized, it's a good time to add in some high-intensity interval training, or HIIT, doing very short bursts of exercise but really going for it. It's a practical way to fit in more activity, with the proven benefit of firing up metabolism without spiking hunger. Try a session or two first thing and you'll feel more energized and burn more fat all day.

A good protocol to follow is Tabata, which is a four-minute round of HIIT. That's right, just four minutes, and you're resting for one-third of it. There are lots of smartphone apps you can download, which will do the timing for you, or you can use a stopwatch. You simply:

- **Exercise for 20 seconds**
- **Rest for 10 seconds**
- **Repeat for a total of eight times (four minutes in total).**

You can choose any exercise but here are some ideas. Try alternating cardio and strength moves.

Cardio
- **Jogging on the spot (or on a rebounder)**
- **Jumping jacks**
- **Side-to-side jumps**
- **Mountain climbers**
- **Burpees**
- **Fast alternate punches, boxing stance**

Strength
- **Squats (without or without a weight held into your chest)**
- **Lunges (with or without hand weights)**
- **Press-ups (full or on knees)**
- **Plank (or alternating side planks)**
- **Sit-ups**
- **Triceps dips (from the edge of the sofa)**

You can do a four-minute round of one exercise for a quick boost – great first thing, before your shower and smoothie. Alternatively, put three or four rounds together, taking a minute's break between each, for a slightly longer but time-efficient workout. We both find Tabata really helps us start the day on a high – we leave home with an extra spring in our step.

Evenings are still a good time for wind-down yoga and stretching, particularly gentle spinal twists which help to massage the gut. Find a good DVD or book, or try one of many online videos or virtual classes.

Time for you

During this phase, find time to create a 'vision board'. You'll need a large noticeboard or piece of card, and lots of pictures from magazines, brochures or newspapers. Over the next nine days, spend a short time each day looking through them and finding pictures that appeal to you and what you'd like for yourself, now and in the future.

We don't mean material possessions or unrealistic bikini-body goals. This is about ideas, symbols and inspiration. What images are you drawn to? What would you like more of in your life? How does healthy and happy feel and look to you?

It could be pictures of delicious, healthy food to represent a way of eating that makes you feel more alive. It could be natural scenes where you'd like to spend more time: forests, beaches, countryside trails. Perhaps a photograph to represent family, a new place to live, or a new career? Maybe a sporting goal or a creative pursuit you'd like to take up? A person you miss who inspires you, a pet that comforts you?

Once you've collected lots of images, arrange and stick them on the board. Then – and here's the important part – place this somewhere you're going to see it *every* day. By your bed is ideal, so your gaze falls on it morning and night whether you're consciously aware of it or not. (Note: you don't want a virtual mood board, because that requires you to turn on a computer to see it. So if you spot something on Pinterest or Instagram that appeals, print it out.)

The idea of a vision board is to speak to your subconscious mind. It helps draw you towards and alert you to things that can help make your dreams a reality. It's less daunting to put together than written goals. It provides a focal point for visualization, rather than a tick list of things to achieve.

There's a wealth of research in favour of visualization as a psychological method for boosting confidence and motivation. It's something Amanda was taught from a young age as a sportsperson and does to this day. And it's done wonders for clients on her wellbeing retreats, too.

	LUNCH	DINNER
DAY 6	Coconut Carrot Soup, with miso stirred through (page 70)	Butternut Squash, Quinoa & Chicken Pot (page 72)
DAY 7	Butternut Squash, Quinoa & Chicken Pot (page 72)	Warming Broth with Vegetables, Noodles & Miso (page 74)
DAY 8	Butternut Squash Salad (page 77)	Pan-fried Tuna, Tofu or Eggs with Green Beans & Lemony Kefir Dressing (page 79)
DAY 9	Pan-fried Tuna, Tofu or Eggs with Green Beans & Lemony Kefir Dressing (page 79)	Spanish Style Chickpeas (page 80)
DAY 10	Shaved Asparagus Salad (page 83)	Super Stir-fry with Miso Soup (page 84)
DAY 11	Super Stir-fry with Miso Soup (page 84)	Pumpkin Soup with Jerusalem Artichokes (page 87)
DAY 12	Pumpkin Soup with Jerusalem Artichokes (page 87)	Turmeric Lentil Bake (page 69)
DAY 13	Green Salad with Turmeric Dressing (page 88)	Warm Grain & Fennel Salad (page 91)
DAY 14	Warm Grain & Fennel Salad (page 91)	Lebanese Lentil Soup (page 93)

PHASE 2 SHOPPING LIST

BREAKFASTS

Replenish the smoothie ingredients from Phase 1 if you need (depending on which you liked/chose), and add the following.

Fresh ingredients

Dairy or coconut kefir
Eggs
Fresh herbs (basil, chives, coriander, parsley)
Kale
Mackerel
Pineapple
Tomatoes
Unsweetened almond milk

Storecupboard ingredients

Chicory root powder
Coconut oil
Raw cacao powder
Raw honey, maple syrup or agave syrup
Seeds (pumpkin, sunflower, flax, chia, hemp, poppy, sesame)
Silken tofu

LUNCHES, DINNERS AND SNACKS

Fresh ingredients

You may already have some of these items left over from Phase 1 – just replenish or substitute as needed.

Apples
Asparagus
Avocados
Bean sprouts
Broccoli
Cabbage
Carrots
Cucumber
Fennel
Fresh basil, coriander, ginger, parsley
Garlic
Green beans
Jerusalem artichokes
Lemons and limes
Mushrooms
Onions and leeks
Pak choi
Peppers
Pumpkin or butternut squash
Red onions
Salad leaves (lettuce, rocket, spinach, watercress)
Spring onions

Swiss chard
Tomatoes (large and cherry)
Chicken breasts
Crème fraîche or natural yogurt
Eggs
Fresh tuna steaks
Kefir
Kimchi
Salmon
Soya milk
Tempeh
Tofu

Storecupboard ingredients

You may already have some of these from Phase 1, so check the cupboards before shopping.

Chickpeas (dried or canned)
Dried basil
Gluten-free oatcakes
Ground spices (cayenne pepper, coriander, cumin, ginger, nutmeg, paprika and turmeric)
Lentils (any, dried or canned)
Miso paste

Nuts for toasting (cashew nuts and almonds)
Olive oil (mild and cold-pressed extra virgin)
Quinoa
Rice noodles
Sauerkraut
Sea salt flakes and black pepper
Seeds for toasting (sesame, pumpkin, sunflower and poppy)
Tahini
Tamari soy sauce
Tomatoes (canned, chopped)
Wholegrain mustard

PHASE 3: REBALANCE

In Phase 3 there are more delicious recipes to try and an even greater diversity of ingredients. There's lots more choice and we're going to reintroduce common gut-irritant foods. Think of this as your decision-making week. You have to be mindful, paying attention to what you're eating and how it makes you feel, then asking, is this good for *me*? It's not about restriction, but freedom.

We've staggered the reintroductions to help you try to identify any which may still be a problem for you.

DAY 15: REINTRODUCING DAIRY

Start small by adding some natural yogurt to your morning smoothie, or crumbled goats' cheese to your soup. Dairy products made from goats' and sheep's milk are generally easier for the body to digest so are a good starting point.

DAY 17: REINTRODUCING GLUTEN

We've started with a slice of rye bread. Rye bread still contains gluten but doesn't contain wheat so it is generally easier to digest. If you have no symptoms with the rye, try adding wheat bread on day 18 or 19 for breakfast or lunch. If you react to that it could be wheat rather than gluten in general that is a problem for you.

DAY 19: REINTRODUCING CHILLI

Chillies are powerful antioxidants and have been shown to boost metabolism to aid weight loss. But in some people they cause heartburn and gut sensitivity. If you know that's you, you can continue to leave out chilli or start mild.

Don't forget to stock up on supplies using the shopping list on page 39, before you get started on this phase.

Phase 3 breakfasts

Continue to start the next seven days with hot water, lemon and optional ginger. You can also continue to enjoy any of the smoothies (*see* page 42), with the optional Phase 2 and/or Phase 3 extras. We've also added some more healthy breakfast ideas for those days when you want something a little different. You can add to those from Phase 2 to give you a selection of healthy breakfasts from which to choose. The recipes for these can be found from page 115.

- **Berry Bircher Muesli (*see* page 55)**
- **Apple & Cinnamon Pancakes (*see* page 56)**
- **Healthy Eggs on Avo Toast (*see* page 58) – from day 17 onwards**

You may also like to try these storecupboard staples for breakfast in a hurry:

- **Gluten-free oat porridge – cooked with non-dairy milk and a drizzle of raw honey or a teaspoon of low-sugar jam.**

Phase 3 lunches and dinners

By now you should have a selection of leftovers in your freezer. There are some new recipes to try in this phase, but if there are days you don't have the time or inclination to cook, simply replace a dish with one of those you batch-cooked earlier in the plan.

Phase 3 puddings and snacks

If you fancy something sweet after a meal, we've included a couple of delicious fruit puddings you could enjoy a few times this week.

- **Berry Banana Bake (*see* page 121)**
- **Stewed Apples with Blueberries (*see* page 122)**

And if you prefer a sweeter snack now, try one of the recipes below.

- **Raw Energy Balls (*see* pages 110–12)**
- **Raw Chocolate Brownies (*see* page 118)**

Phase 3 drinks

If you are happy sticking with water, herbal and green tea, chicory coffee and kombucha, keep it up. You can reintroduce tea and coffee now if you like, but don't undo your good work and exceed two cups of coffee or two or three cups of tea a day. Ideally have them before 2pm so the caffeine doesn't interfere with sleep. A little milk is fine but steer clear of coffee shop sizes and very milky and creamy coffees. Sugar and syrups are still off limits and you'd probably find them sickly now anyway.

You can, if you like, indulge in the odd tipple during Phase 3 – that's right, we're reintroducing alcohol for those who want it. Just limit yourself to one or two 125ml (4fl oz) glasses of wine (ideally red) over the week.

How you might feel during Phase 3

Hopefully you're feeling full of vitality and motivated to continue by seeing the results you have achieved so far. Most people find they have lost several pounds by now. They're feeling slimmer, with a flatter tummy, and have often lost a couple of inches or more from their waist. That's what you get when you're not relying on sugar, alcohol and processed foods.

The interesting part of this phase is seeing how your body reacts when we introduce some of the food types you haven't had for the past fortnight. You may not have thought you were sensitive to anything, but once they become 'new' to you again, it's easier to see exactly what effect they have.

Please note that this phase – and the G Plan in general – isn't about tellling you to cut things out unnecessarily. There's no need to fear any foods. Often we are intolerant to things in large amounts. When your diet lacks diversity it's easy to overdo foods like wheat and dairy without realizing. The chances are you can still enjoy everything, but it pays to be aware if some items should be avoided, or kept to small portions or occasional treats.

Maintaining your food diary during this phase is crucial, so you can track any symptoms. Note if you feel bloated, have stomach pains, if your bowel movements change significantly, if you feel more tired or suffer from brain fog, get a runny nose or other respiratory symptoms, these could all be signs of intolerance.

Keep active

Did you know your body adapts quickly to regular exercise? It becomes more efficient as you get stronger and fitter. So the activity gets easier – but body changes will start to plateau.

There's an easy way to overcome this: add as much variety to your workouts as there now is in your diet. So long as you shake things up every few weeks, upping the duration or intensity of an activity, you'll continue to get results. More importantly, you won't get bored.

Keeping active for life is about so much more than going to the gym, riding your bike or strapping on an activity tracker to count your steps (although those things are all great). What about stand-up paddle-boarding, aerial yoga, circus skills or tap dancing? Why not?

Pledge to try something new once a month and you'll keep the 'fresh and exciting' quota high. Maybe there's something on your vision board to inspire you? Ask yourself the following questions to help steer you towards some new activities to try – but don't be afraid to go outside your comfort zone, too.

- **Do I prefer to exercise in the mornings or the evenings?**
- **Do I like to be outdoors or inside?**
- **Am I happier exercising on my own or with others?**
- **Would I prefer to be taught or learn by myself?**
- **Would I like to meet some new people or catch up with old friends?**
- **Do I want to get wet and muddy or stay warm and dry?**
- **Do I prefer uplifting music or quiet contemplation?**

Time for you

If you're still practising the belly breathing relaxation technique from Phase 1, keep it up. You might like to take meditation to the next level; it's a valuable skill but can feel daunting if you don't know what to do.

There are lots of different techniques and you'll find some easier than others. Some people like to simply observe where they are and how they feel.

Others repeat a mantra to themselves or chant. Others may gaze at a candle or use visualization. It's worth finding a local meditation class or teacher, or a yoga class that incorporates meditation. There are even smartphone apps and CDs that talk you through daily meditations you can do any place, anywhere.

You don't need to invest lots of time in meditation, sessions of 10–15 minutes are fine. But when it comes to reducing stress – so important for digestive health – and increasing productivity, it's time well spent.

	LUNCH	DINNER
DAY 15	Lebanese Lentil Soup, topped with crumbled goats' cheese (page 93)	Warming Broth with Vegetables, Noodles & Miso, and protein of your choice (page 74)
DAY 16	Kale & Avocado Salad (page 94)	Cauli-Pizza (page 97)
DAY 17	Rocket, Walnut & Beetroot Salad with Gorgonzola (page 99)	Asparagus Soup with rye toast (page 100)
DAY 18	Asparagus Soup with rye toast (page 100)	Vegetable Frittata with green salad (page 103)
DAY 19	Vegetable Frittata with green salad (page 103)	Chilli Con Carne with brown rice (page 104)
DAY 20	Chilli Con Carne with spinach, avocado and a wholemeal wrap (page 104)	Garlic Prawns with Quinoa Salad (page 106)
DAY 21	Quinoa Salad with toasted seeds and hard-boiled egg (page 106)	Stuffed Peppers with Marinated Salmon or Chicken (page 109)

PHASE 3 SHOPPING LIST

BREAKFASTS

Replenish the recipe ingredients from Phases 1 and 2 if you need (depending on which you liked/chose) and, if needed, add the following.

Fresh ingredients

Apples
Greek or live natural yogurt
Lemons
Mushrooms
Spring onions

Storecupboard ingredients

Almonds
Medjool dates or dried figs
Rye bread
White wine vinegar

LUNCHES, DINNERS AND SNACKS

Fresh ingredients

You may already have some of these ingredients left over from Phases 1 and 2 – just replenish or substitute as needed.

Apples
Asparagus
Avocados
Bananas
Beetroot (raw or cooked)
Berries (fresh or frozen)
Blueberries (fresh or frozen)
Broccoli
Carrots
Cauliflower
Courgettes
Fresh basil, coriander, ginger, mint, parsley
Jerusalem artichokes
Garlic
Kale
Lemons and limes
Mushrooms
New potatoes
Onions
Oranges
Pears
Red peppers
Rocket
Sprouted seeds
Tomatoes (large, cherry)
Spinach and watercress
Almond milk
Butter
Chicken breasts
Eggs
Feta cheese
Goats' cheese

Good-quality minced steak or turkey
Gorgonzola
Greek or natural yogurt
Mozzarella balls
Parmesan
Prawns
Salmon
Tempeh
Tofu

Storecupboard ingredients

Again, check your cupboards as you may have some of these ingredients left from Phases 1 and 2.

Almonds (whole, flaked and ground)
Brazil nuts
Brown rice (dry or steam pouches)
Buckwheat
Cashew nuts
Chickpeas (canned)
Chilli powder
Cocoa powder (raw)
Coconut (oil, desiccated, flakes and flour)
Dried apricots
Gluten-free oats and oatcakes

Ground spices (cardamon, cinnamon, cloves, cumin, ginger, nutmeg, paprika and turmeric)
Harissa chilli paste
Honey (raw, set and Manuka)
Kimchi
Lentils (canned)
Low-sugar jam (optional)
Medjool dates
Miso paste
Mixed beans (canned)
Olive oil (mild and cold-pressed extra virgin)
Pecan nuts
Pine nuts
Pitted black olives
Quinoa
Sea salt flakes and black pepper
Seeds (flax, sesame, chia and hemp)
Sauerkraut
Spirulina
Tomatoes (canned and chopped, purée and passata)
Unsweetened peanut butter
Vegetable stock
Walnuts

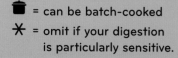 = can be batch-cooked

✳ = omit if your digestion
is particularly sensitive.

THE RECIPES

BREAKFASTS

THE SMOOTHIES

You can use fresh or frozen fruit in the smoothie recipes below. Freeze peeled bananas in slices or halves to use throughout the plan. This will ensure you always have bananas to hand and is a great way to make best use of any that are going slightly brown. Frozen bananas also add a nice chill to a smoothie, or you could add crushed ice, if you prefer.

To make the smoothies, place all the ingredients in a blender and add your chosen liquid. Dairy-free milks, such as coconut or almond milk, are good choices, or you could use coconut water or plain water to thin your smoothie to the desired consistency. You can always add a little more liquid if it turns out too thick after blending.

PHASE 1: Stick to the core ingredients listed for each smoothie.

PHASES 2 AND 3: You can use the same core recipes but we've given you some optional add-ins to mix up the flavours and textures.

Don't be tempted to add your own natural sweeteners, unless the recipe says you can use raw honey (from Phase 3 in some recipes). We know both sugar and artificial sweeteners are bad news for gut bacteria. But it's also thought that natural alternatives, such as agave, xylitol and stevia, can disrupt the microbiome – not to mention keep up your dependence on sweet flavours. If you really feel you need sweetness, a tiny squeeze in one of these super-healthy smoothies isn't going to negate all the benefits, but do try without first.

The berries add a vitamin C hit to support your immune function, while the oats will help fill you up on busy mornings.

Rich in healthy fats, the avocado gives this smoothie a creamy texture. This is a thick, filling smoothie so add more water if you need to make it easier to drink.

Berry Banana

1 SERVING

2 tablespoons mixed berries, fresh or frozen
½ banana
150ml (¼ pint) non-dairy milk, coconut water or water
1 tablespoon gluten-free oats

PHASE 2: Replace some or all of the liquid with probiotic-rich kefir. Choose either a dairy or coconut kefir (*see* page 19).

PHASE 3: Replace some or all of the liquid with kefir, as above, or swap for natural or Greek yogurt for an extra protein boost. Make sure you buy real Greek yogurt not 'Greek-style yogurt', and avoid low-fat or flavoured products. Check the ingredients list – it should only contain pasteurized milk and live and active bacterial cultures (*see* page 18).

Avo Banana

1 SERVING

1 small ripe avocado
1 small banana
150ml (¼ pint) non-dairy milk, coconut water or water
1 teaspoon ground cinnamon

PHASE 2: Add extra fibre with a handful of spinach or kale. Replace some or all of the liquid with probiotic-rich kefir.

PHASE 3: Swap the cinnamon for a little raw honey or vanilla extract for a sweeter hit, if you like.

Chia seeds are rich in omega-3, which is great at reducing inflammation and supporting your gut lining. Add them to your smoothie last, just before blending, or you'll find they turn gelatinous on contact with the milk and are a pain to get out of the blender!

Adding tofu to a smoothie may sound odd, but it gives a great texture and provides valuable protein to support gut repair.

Blueberry Chia

1 SERVING

1 small banana
1 handful of blueberries, fresh or frozen
150ml (¼ pint) non-dairy milk, coconut water or water
1 teaspoon desiccated coconut
2 tablespoons chia seeds (black, white or a mixture)

PHASE 2: Bulk up your smoothie and add extra fibre with 1 tablespoon gluten-free oats and mix in some kefir for valuable probiotics.

PHASE 3: Add 1 tablespoon natural or Greek yogurt to boost the protein level of this smoothie.

Protein Punch

1 SERVING

1 handful of berries of your choice, fresh or frozen
1 small banana
1 lime, peeled and deseeded
25g (1oz) silken tofu (about ½ block)
150ml (¼ pint) non-dairy milk, coconut water or water

PHASE 2: Replace some or all of the liquid with probiotic-rich kefir.

PHASE 3: Push up the protein and fibre levels by adding 1 handful of almonds (soaked in cold water for a minimum of 4 hours) and 1 handful of spinach or kale.

Flaxseeds are high in omega-3 and a great source of insoluble fibre to keep your bowels moving. Leave out the flax if your stomach is extra sensitive. Freeze the remaining papaya and banana for use in the Tropical Treat Smoothie (see page 47) another day.

A healthy protein source, nuts also provide fibre and good fats to balance mood.

Go with the Flow

1 SERVING

½ papaya, cut into chunks
4 strawberries
½ banana
150ml (¼ pint) non-dairy milk, coconut water or water
1 teaspoon flaxseeds *
5–6 mint leaves

PHASE 2: Swap the strawberries for some digestive enzyme-boosting pineapple.

PHASE 3: Add some extra fibre with 1 handful of spinach or kale, and extra protein by adding 2 tablespoons of natural or Greek yogurt.

Nuts About Nutrition

1 SERVING

1 small banana
1 tablespoon Almond Butter (*see* page 115)
1 tablespoon gluten-free oats
1 teaspoon ground cinnamon
150ml (¼ pint) non-dairy milk, coconut water or water

PHASE 2: Replace some or all of the liquid with probiotic-rich kefir.

PHASE 3: Give your nuts some chocolate flavour by adding 1 teaspoon raw cacao powder and a little raw honey or vanilla.

The omega-3 in the flaxseeds and the curcumin in the turmeric provide valuable anti-inflammatory effects in the body.

Adding greens and spirulina to your smoothie will provide valuable magnesium and B vitamins, which will help boost energy.

Replenish

1 SERVING

½ small banana
1 heaped teaspoon flaxseeds*
½ teaspoon ground cinnamon
pinch of ground turmeric
150ml (¼ pint) non-dairy milk, coconut water or water

PHASE 2: Replace some or all of the liquid with probiotic-rich kefir.

PHASE 3: Add a touch of sweetness with some raw honey, if you like.

Green Goodness

1 SERVING

1 handful of spinach
1 small ripe banana
150ml (¼ pint) non-dairy milk,
    coconut water or water
1 tablespoon chia seeds
1 teaspoon spirulina*

PHASE 2: Add some probiotic-boosting kefir and boost your healthy fats by adding ½ avocado, or add some pineapple to help boost your digestive enzymes.

PHASE 3: Add some Greek yogurt and a touch of sweetness with 2 Medjool dates, if you wish.

Need a little help getting going in the morning? This smoothie provides a balanced level of caffeine and spice to pep you up without needing to head to the coffee shop.

Kickstarter

1 SERVING

1 small banana
100ml (3½fl oz) brewed and cooled green tea
  or matcha tea
½ lemon, peeled and deseeded
pinch of cayenne pepper*
6 mint leaves

PHASE 2: Add a dash of kefir for probiotics and a creamy texture.

PHASE 3: Add a dried fig or Medjool date for extra sweetness, if you like.

The papaya in this smoothie provides digestive enzymes, while the ginger is soothing. You could replace half the liquid with light coconut milk for extra creaminess, if you prefer. Use the papaya chunks and banana saved from your Go with the Flow smoothie (see page 45).

Tropical Treat

1 SERVING

½ papaya, cut into chunks and frozen
½ banana, frozen
150ml (¼ pint) non-dairy milk, coconut water or water
1 teaspoon grated fresh root ginger*
lime juice, to taste
seeds and flesh of 1 passion fruit (optional)

PHASE 2: Add some pineapple to further boost your digestive enzymes. Replace some or all of the liquid with probiotic-rich kefir.

PHASE 3: Add extra protein with some Greek yogurt and a dash of kefir for probiotics.

This recipe makes one pot, but you can make multiple portions and stash them in the refrigerator for an easy 'grab-and-go' breakfast. Cinnamon contains chromium, a trace mineral which can help balance blood sugar and prevent sugar cravings. You can substitute up to half the liquid with kefir, if you like.

Coconut Cinnamon Chia Pot

PHASE 2 ONWARDS

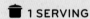 **1 SERVING**

40g (1½oz) chia seeds
½ teaspoon ground cinnamon
2 teaspoons desiccated coconut
200–250ml (7–9fl oz) coconut or
    almond milk

OPTIONAL EXTRAS:
sunflower or pumpkin seeds
fresh berries

Place the chia in a small bowl, tumbler or jar and add the cinnamon and desiccated coconut.

Pour on the milk, stir well and set aside for 10–15 minutes until the chia has soaked up the liquid.

Serve as it is or top with seeds and/or berries. The pots can be covered with clingfilm or a lid and stored in the refrigerator for up to 3 days.

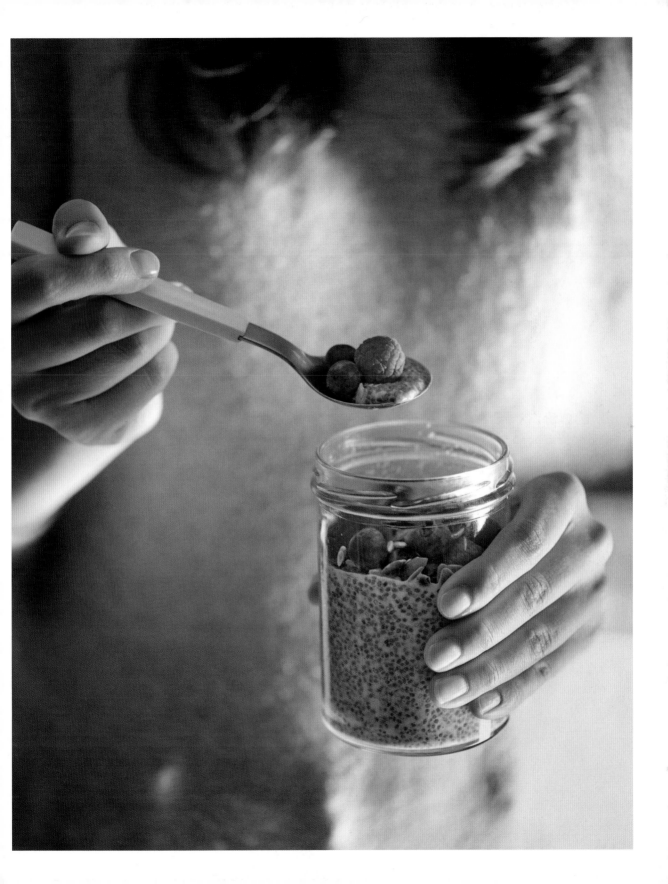

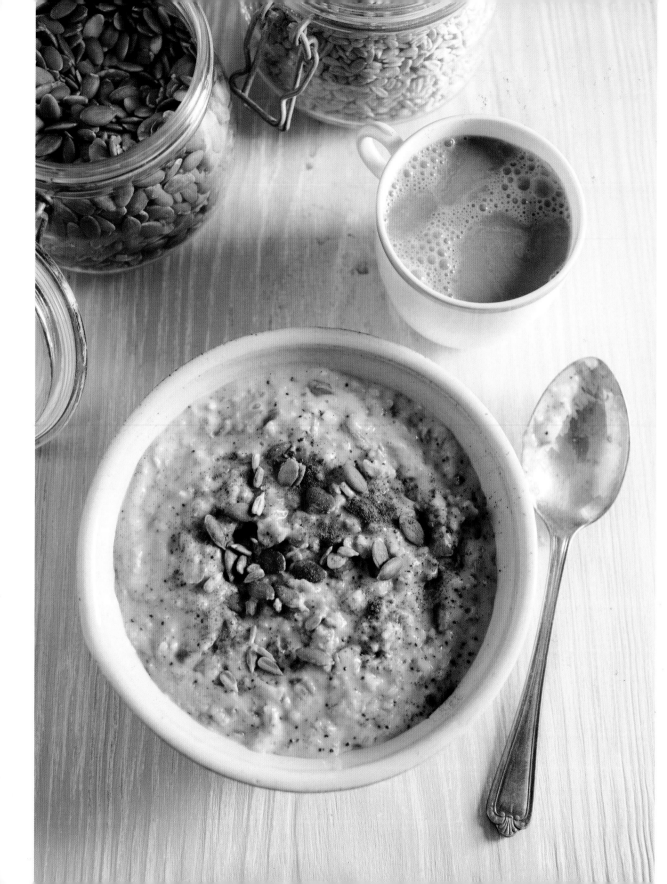

The seeds in this dish ensure it keeps you feeling full until lunchtime.

Don't worry, this isn't a breakfast in itself, but an additional drink option which you can enjoy from Phase 2 onwards. Chicory root is a fantastic prebiotic and tastes remarkably like coffee. Give it a go.

Mixed Seed Porridge

PHASE 2 ONWARDS

1 SERVING

70g (2½oz) gluten-free porridge oats
50g (1¾oz) mixed seeds, such as pumpkin, sunflower, flax, chia, hemp, poppy, sesame
250–500ml (9–18fl oz) almond, coconut or oat milk
½ teaspoon ground cinnamon

Place all the ingredients in a saucepan over a medium heat, mix well then heat gently until bubbling and thickened.

Chicory Root 'Coffee'

PHASE 2 ONWARDS

1 SERVING

1 mugful of non-dairy milk
1 tablespoon organic roasted chicory root powder
1 tablespoon raw cacao powder
dash of raw honey, maple or agave syrup, or another natural sweetener (optional)

Heat the milk until hot but not boiling. Stir in the chicory root and cacao. Add a squeeze of sweetener to taste, only if needed.

An alternative cooked breakfast, this dish is rich in healthy fats, which support heart health. Cooking tomatoes helps to release the antioxidant lycopene, which protects your body from free radicals.

Healthy Cooked Breakfast

PHASE 2 ONWARDS

1 SERVING

2 large or 6 small tomatoes, halved
1 teaspoon coconut oil (optional)
chopped fresh herbs, such as
    coriander, basil, chives, parsley
1 large handful of spinach leaves
½ avocado, sliced
sea salt flakes and pepper, to taste

PROTEIN OF YOUR CHOICE:

2 fresh mackerel fillets (about
    100g/3½ oz)
100g (3½ oz) silken tofu (about ½ a
    block), sliced
or 2 eggs, beaten

Preheat the oven to 200°C (400°F), Gas Mark 6. Place the tomato halves, cut sides up, in an ovenproof dish and bake for 10–15 minutes until softened.

If using mackerel, cook under a preheated hot grill, skin side up, for about 5 minutes until cooked through.

If using tofu, heat the coconut oil in a frying pan and cook the tofu until golden on both sides.

If using eggs, heat the coconut oil in a small saucepan, add the eggs and heat gently until scrambled and cooked.

Sprinkle your choice of protein with the chopped herbs and serve with the tomatoes, spinach and avocado, seasoned with salt and pepper.

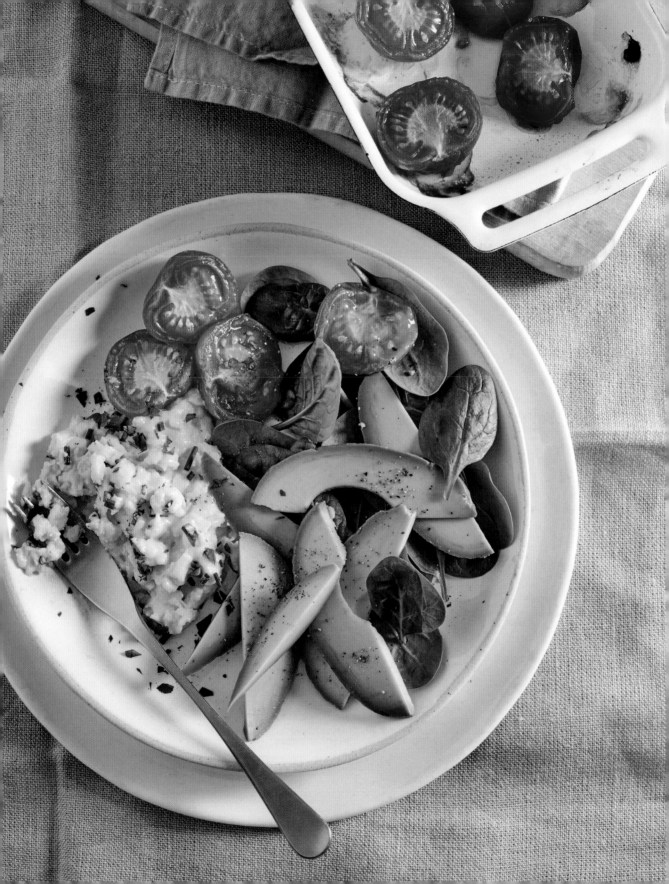

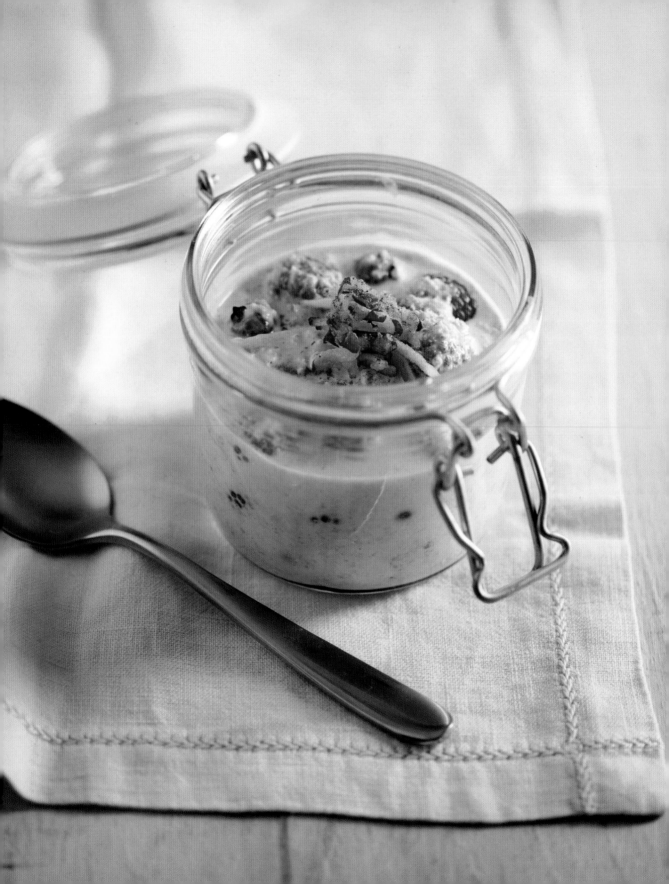

A simple, nourishing and filling breakfast which can be prepared in advance, ready for you to grab-and-go in the morning.

Berry Bircher Muesli

 1 SERVING

70g (2½oz) gluten-free oats
250ml (9fl oz) coconut or almond
   milk
handful of blueberries, raspberries
   or strawberries

OPTIONAL EXTRAS:
1 teaspoon desiccated coconut
dusting of ground cinnamon
generous spoonful of live natural
   yogurt
1 tablespoon kefir
grated apple

Place all the ingredients in a bowl, mix well and leave to soak for 15 minutes or overnight. Add any of the optional extras you like, and tuck in.

Apples contain a natural fibre called pectin, which helps feed the probiotic-friendly bacteria in your gut. If you need a sweetener (and you may not, the cinnamon, banana and apple keep these naturally sweet), use natural maple syrup – sparingly – as it's been shown to cause fewer problems with digestion and also contains beneficial antioxidant and anti-inflammatory compounds. Both coconut and almond oil can be found in most supermarkets, but you can use a knob of fresh butter instead. All these fats are stable at high temperatures so are safer to cook with.

Apple & Cinnamon Pancakes   PHASE 3 ONWARDS

2–3 SERVINGS

2 apples, peeled and cut into chunks
juice of ½ lemon
1 teaspoon ground cinnamon, plus
    extra for the apples (optional)
90g (3¼oz) gluten-free oats
55g (2oz) blanched almonds
250ml (9fl oz) almond milk
1 banana
coconut or almond oil, for greasing

TO SERVE:
drizzle of maple syrup (optional)
natural yogurt (optional)

Place the apples in a small saucepan with the lemon juice and a dash of water and cook gently for 5–10 minutes until softened. Add a pinch of cinnamon to taste, if you like.

Blend the oats and nuts in a blender or food processor until a fine flour forms, then add the milk, banana and cinnamon. Continue to blend to form a batter.

Grease a frying pan with oil and set over a medium heat. Pour about one-sixth of the batter into the pan and cook for 2–3 minutes until the mixture sets. Flip the pancake and cook on the other side until golden. Repeat to make 6 pancakes.

Serve the pancakes topped with the apple, with a drizzle of maple syrup if needed, and a spoonful of yogurt, if you like.

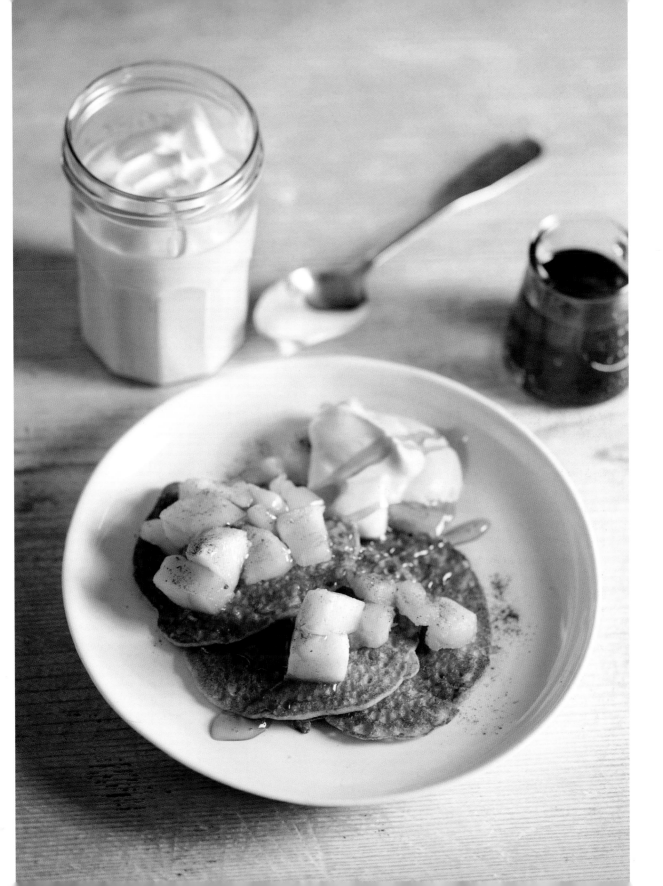

This recipe can be introduced from day 17 onwards. Eggs are a great protein source and the rye bread used here is gentler on your digestion than wheat bread.

Healthy Eggs on Avo Toast

PHASE 3 ONWARDS

1 SERVING

2 tablespoons white wine vinegar
2 eggs
½ avocado, mashed
2 slices of rye bread, toasted
½ handful of spinach, chopped
sea salt flakes and pepper

Place a small saucepan of water over a medium heat, add the vinegar and bring to the boil. Lower the heat so the water is just simmering.

Crack the eggs into 2 small cups or ramekins then gently lower the eggs into the water. Poach for 2–3 minutes, depending on how soft you like your eggs.

Spread the mashed avocado on the rye toast and top with the chopped spinach and eggs. Season with salt and pepper to serve.

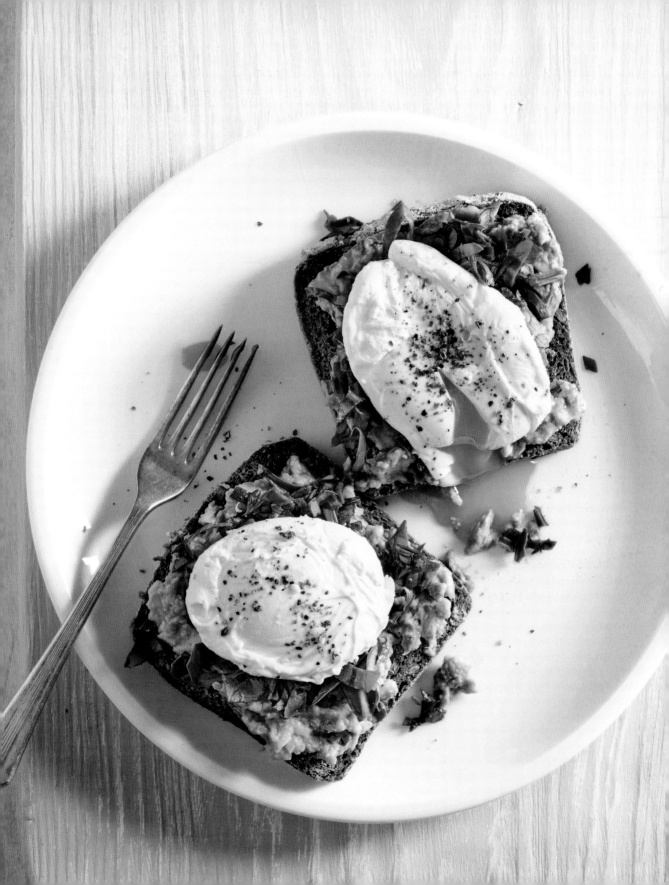

LUNCHES & DINNERS

Making your own stock means you know exactly what's in your food. Otherwise, buy an organic, low-salt version.

You can make vegetable or chicken stock. Collagen and glucosamine in chicken stock strengthens your gut lining. The acidity of the apple cider vinegar helps to draw out the minerals and goodness from the bones.

Homemade Stock

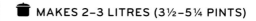 **MAKES 2–3 LITRES (3½–5¼ PINTS)**

3–4 litres (5¼–7 pints) water
6 carrots, chopped
6 celery sticks, including leafy ends, chopped
2 onions, chopped
4 bay leaves
1 chicken carcass, cooked or raw (optional)
2 tablespoons apple cider vinegar (optional)

For vegetable stock: Pour the measured water into your largest saucepan (preferably stainless steel) and add the vegetables immediately after chopping them. Add the bay leaves and bring to the boil. Reduce the heat and simmer for a minimum of 45 minutes.

For chicken stock: Follow the instructions above, but add the chicken carcass and apple cider vinegar to the vegetables and simmer for a minimum of 3 hours. Remove from the heat, allow to cool, then strain the stock. Store in a sealed container for up to 1 week in the refrigerator or up to 3 months in the freezer. If freezing, store in small pots for easy portion control.

A simple cleansing and warming broth which provides valuable minerals and amino acids (proteins) to support your gut health and immunity. Coconut milk makes this incredibly filling and contains a type of saturated fat that can be healthy in small amounts (see page 23). Add chicken, salmon, tofu or tempeh to this dish for a boost of protein.

This recipe makes four portions of basic broth, so set aside half of the broth before adding the remaining ingredients to the dish and store it in the freezer for Phase 2. Half the remaining finished dish can be saved for lunch tomorrow.

Warming Broth

🍲 MAKES 2 SERVINGS

800ml (27fl oz) vegetable or
   chicken stock (*see* page 60)
800ml (27fl oz) coconut milk
4 tablespoons lemon juice
1 teaspoon finely grated lemon zest
3–4 teaspoons finely grated fresh
   root ginger*
2 garlic* cloves, crushed
3–4 teaspoons Chinese five spice
   powder*
4 kaffir lime leaves (optional)
125g (4½oz) spinach, shredded
handful of chopped fresh coriander,
   plus extra to garnish
sea salt flakes and pepper

YOUR CHOICE OF PROTEIN, ABOUT 100G (3½OZ):

chicken
salmon
tofu, cubed
or tempeh, cubed

If using chicken or salmon, preheat the oven to 180°C (350°F), Gas Mark 4. Place the chicken or salmon in an ovenproof dish, cover and bake the chicken for 25 minutes or the salmon for 15 minutes, or until cooked through. Slice, then set aside.

Place the stock, coconut milk, lemon juice, lemon zest, ginger, garlic, five spice and lime leaves, if using, in a large saucepan over a high heat and bring to the boil. Reduce the heat and simmer for 5 minutes.

Set aside three-quarters of the liquid, one portion for tomorrow, and the other portions to be frozen for Phase 2, removing the lime leaves, if used, before freezing.

Add the spinach and coriander to the remaining broth, with the tofu or tempeh, if using. Bring to the boil and simmer for 3–5 minutes.

Season to taste, remove any remaining lime leaves and serve in a deep bowl, topped with the chicken or salmon, if using. Garnish with a little extra coriander.

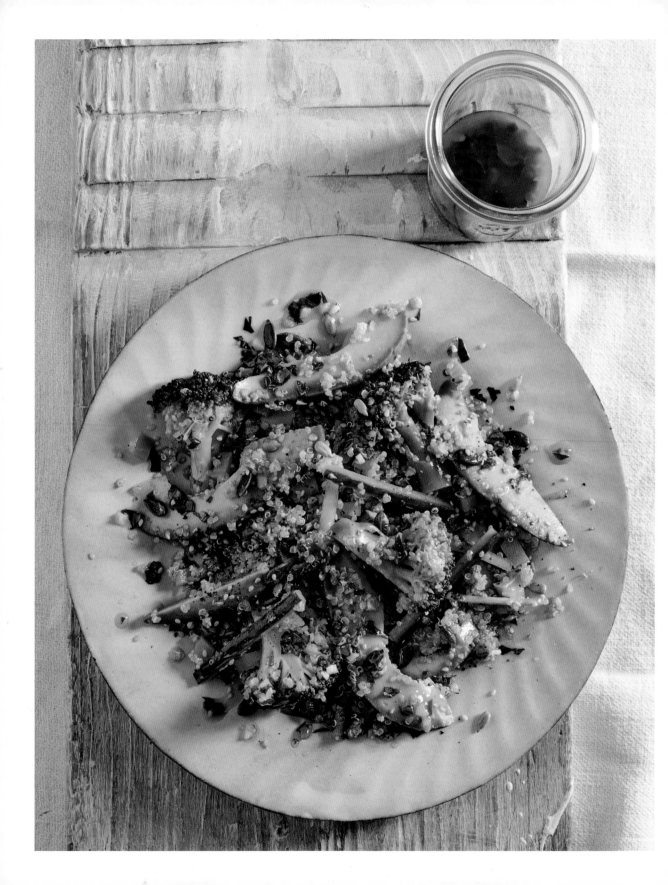

Used like a grain, quinoa is actually an ancient seed and provides protein and complex carbohydrates which help you to feel full and sustain balanced energy levels. As well as being available as a dry grain, quinoa also comes in steam pouches to save time. Don't forget to save half the cooked quinoa for lunch on day 3. You also need to save half the toasted seeds in an airtight container for lunch on day 2; and save half the dressing in an airtight container in the refrigerator for dinner on day 3.

Quinoa Salad with Pesto Dressing & Toasted Seeds

DAY 1

 1 SERVING

125g (4½oz) dry quinoa, rinsed
60g (2¼oz) mixed seeds, such as
   sesame, pumpkin, sunflower
1 carrot, diced
4 large broccoli florets, halved
½ cucumber, cut into matchsticks
½ avocado, sliced

DRESSING:
3 tablespoons extra virgin olive oil
3 tablespoons lemon juice
2 tablespoons finely chopped basil
2 garlic* cloves, finely chopped
sea salt flakes and pepper

Whisk the dressing ingredients together until well combined, season lightly and set aside to infuse.

Cook the quinoa according to the packet instructions.

Place the seeds in a dry frying pan over a medium heat for 3–4 minutes, stirring frequently, until lightly toasted.

Cook the carrot and broccoli in a steamer over a saucepan of gently simmering water until just tender.

Place half the quinoa, all of the vegetables, half the seeds, the cucumber and the avocado in a bowl with half of the dressing, toss to combine and serve warm. Alternatively, leave to cool and mix together just before serving if you'd prefer.

Store the remaining quinoa and dressing in two airtight containers in the refrigerator and the remaining toasted seeds in an airtight jar for later use.

Ginger is not only delicious, it's warming and can help lower inflammation in the gut, too. Use a selection of different vegetables for this casserole – whatever you have in the refrigerator. Swede, carrots, parsnips, turnips, pumpkin or butternut squash, celeriac, leek, fennel and celery are all good choices. Set aside half the finished dish for lunch tomorrow.

Vegetable & Ginger Casserole

DAYS 2 & 3

2 SERVINGS

400ml (14fl oz) vegetable or chicken stock (*see* page 60)
1 teaspoon smoked paprika*
½ teaspoon dried thyme
2 garlic* cloves, crushed
800g (1lb 12oz) mixed vegetables, cut into large chunks
2cm (¾ inch) fresh root ginger*, grated
sea salt flakes and pepper
1 tablespoon finely chopped fresh coriander, to garnish

YOUR CHOICE OF PROTEIN, ABOUT 200G (7OZ):
chicken drumsticks or thighs
white fish
or tofu

Preheat the oven to 200°C (400°F), Gas Mark 6.

Place the stock, paprika, thyme and garlic in a large casserole dish, season to taste and stir well. Add the vegetables and ginger and bake, covered, for 1¼ hours.

If using chicken, lightly brown the meat in a frying pan over a high heat, then add it to the casserole after 35 minutes of cooking.

If using white fish or tofu, cut them into chunks and add to the casserole after it has been cooking for 1 hour.

Serve half the casserole in a bowl, sprinkled with the coriander, then set the remainder aside and store in an airtight container in the refrigerator overnight.

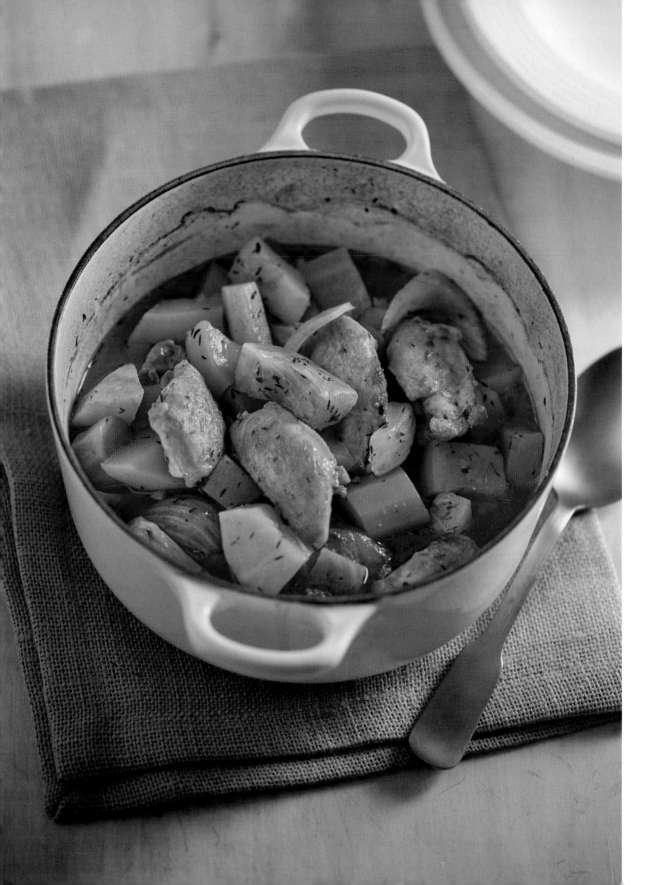

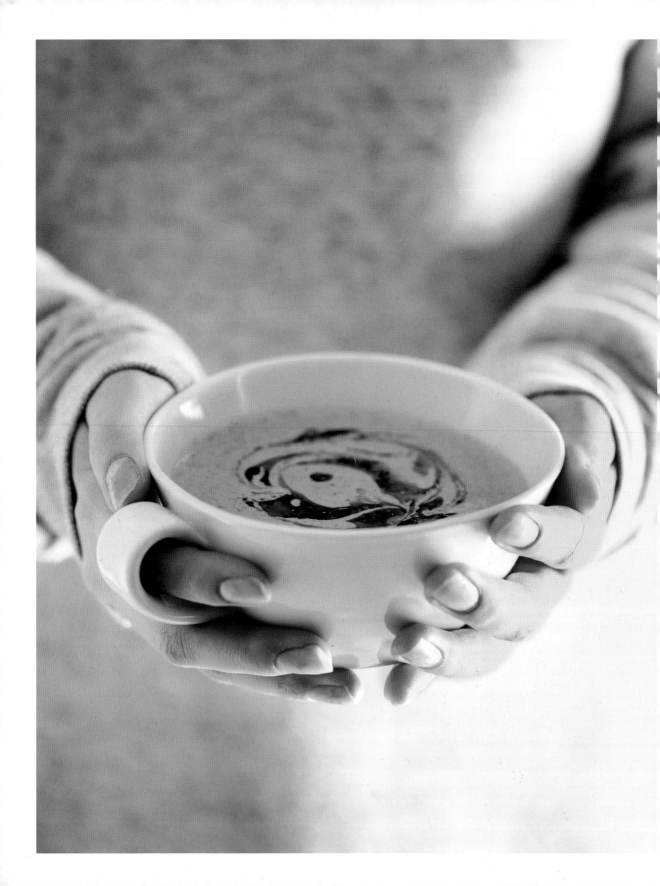

Broccoli is known as a cruciferous vegetable, packed with nutrients that support your liver and aid detoxification. This recipe makes two portions, half for today, and the other half for lunch tomorrow.

Creamy Broccoli Pesto Soup

DAYS 3 & 4

2 SERVINGS

1 head of broccoli, stem and all, roughly chopped
1 litre (1¾ pints) water
leftover pesto dressing from lunch on day 1 (*see* page 63)
125g (4½oz) cashew nuts, soaked for 1–2 hours in cold water and drained
sea salt flakes and pepper
lemon wedges, to serve

Place the broccoli, measured water and all but 1 tablespoon of the pesto dressing in a large saucepan over a high heat and bring to the boil. Reduce the heat and simmer gently for about 10–12 minutes until the broccoli is tender.

Add the nuts and season to taste, then blend until smooth using a hand-held blender or a food processor, adding more water if the consistency is too thick.

Serve half the soup with a squeeze of lemon juice and ½ tablespoon of reserved pesto dressing drizzled over. Set the remainder aside and store in an airtight container in the refrigerator overnight.

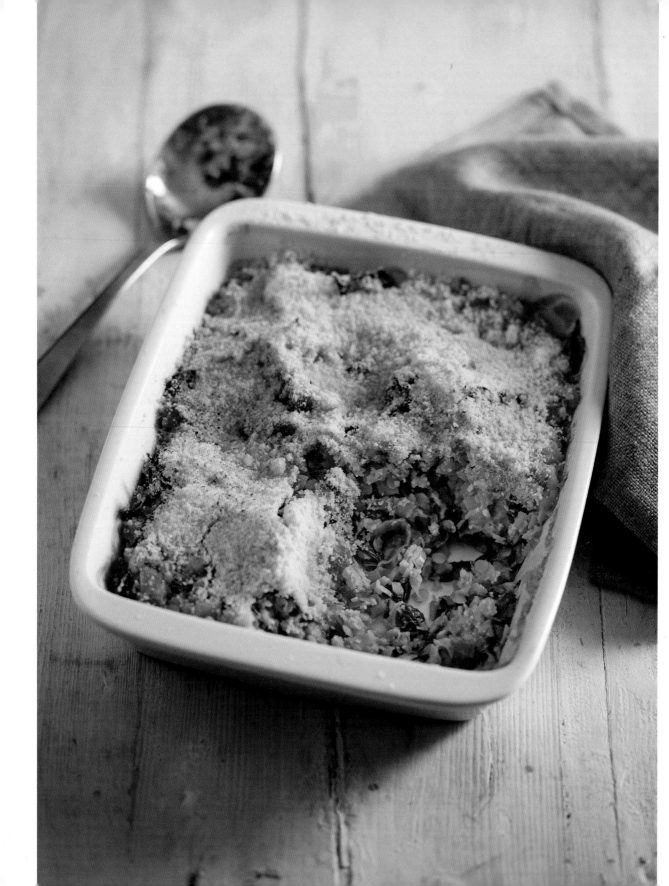

People often struggle to digest lentils and they're thought to cause bloating and excess wind. However, if prepared properly, they shouldn't cause digestive issues and are a great source of vegetable protein and fibre, which keeps you feeling fuller for longer and helps to keep your digestive tract moving.

We're introducing all legumes slowly in this plan to avoid any adverse digestive reactions. When using lentils or beans, soak them and wash thoroughly to remove anti-nutrients called phytates, or phytic acid. This will make them easier to digest and helps to prevent mineral loss (as the presence of phytates weakens your absorption of zinc, calcium and iron). Even if you're using canned lentils, ensure you rinse off the white froth as it can still contain phytic acid.

This recipe makes four portions. Eat one today, save one for tomorrow and freeze the other portions for a quick dinner later in the plan. If you make it again, try using different green vegetables: it's delicious with chard or asparagus, too.

Turmeric Lentil Bake

DAYS 4, 5 & 12

4 SERVINGS

2 tablespoons olive oil
1 garlic* clove, crushed
2 celery sticks, chopped
1 leek, sliced
2 carrots, chopped
½ teaspoon dried thyme
1 teaspoon grated fresh root ginger*
½ teaspoon ground turmeric*
225g (8oz) dried red lentils, soaked in cold water for 1–2 hours, or 800g (1lb 12oz) canned lentils, rinsed and drained
600ml (20fl oz) water or vegetable stock (*see page 60*)
200g (7oz) spinach
50g (1¾oz) ground almonds
sea salt flakes and pepper

Heat the oil in a large saucepan over a low heat and add the garlic. Sweat gently for 1–2 minutes until softened, then add the celery, leek, carrots, herbs and spices.

If using dried lentils, rinse them well, then add to the pan with the water or stock and stir through. Increase the heat and bring to the boil, then reduce the heat and simmer for about 20 minutes until the lentils are soft and the water has been absorbed.

Meanwhile, preheat the oven to 200°C (400°F), Gas Mark 6.

Stir in the spinach and canned lentils, if using, season to taste, then transfer the mixture to an ovenproof dish. Top with the ground almonds, then bake for 20 minutes, or until the topping is golden. Divide the bake into four portions and enjoy one now. Store one leftover portion in an airtight container in the refrigerator overnight, and freeze the other two portions separately.

Carrots are rich in vitamin A, which supports gut health and immune function. Don't forget to save half of the soup for lunch tomorrow when you can serve it with a teaspoon of miso stirred through.

Coconut Carrot Soup

DAYS 5 & 6

🍲 **2 SERVINGS**

4 carrots, about 300g (10½oz), chopped

4cm (1½ inches) fresh root ginger*, chopped

300ml (½ pint) almond milk

250ml (9fl oz) coconut milk

½ teaspoon ground turmeric

½ teaspoon ground cumin*

½ teaspoon sea salt flakes

a squeeze of lime juice

TO SERVE:

chopped fresh coriander

yogurt or ¼ avocado, chopped

Place the carrots and ginger in a large saucepan with the milks and bring to the boil over a medium heat. Reduce the heat and simmer for 10–15 minutes until the carrots are tender.

Remove from the heat, add the spices and salt then blend until smooth using a hand-held blender or a food processor.

Pour the soup back into the saucepan to reheat if needed. Squeeze in some lime juice to taste and add more liquid, if necessary, to reach the desired consistency.

Serve half the soup garnished with yogurt or chopped avocado and fresh coriander. Set the remaining soup aside and store in an airtight container in the refrigerator overnight.

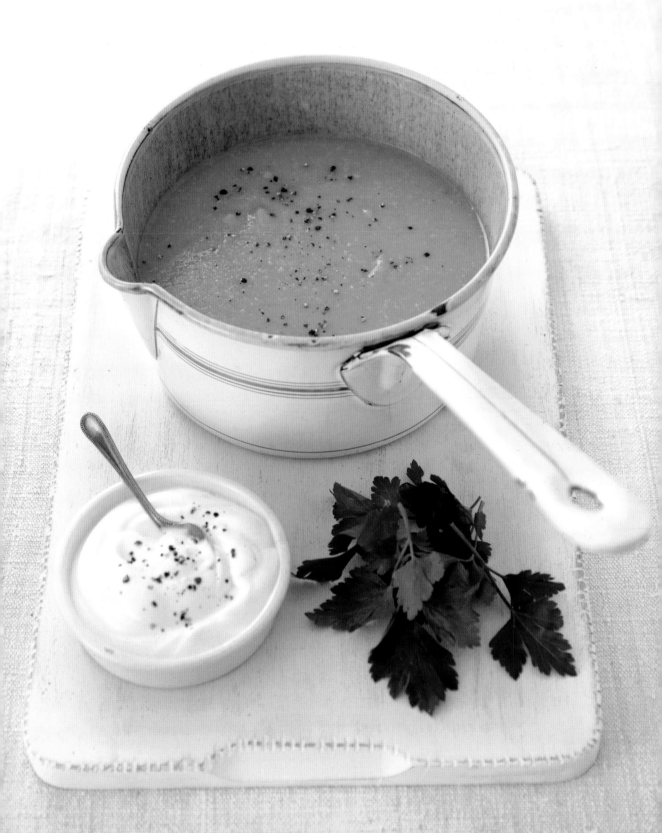

A simple, hearty and filling meal which is rich in gut- and mood-boosting proteins. The chicken can be replaced by chickpeas, if you prefer. This recipe makes two or three portions: save some for lunch tomorrow, and freeze a portion for later in the plan if you have any leftovers. Save one-quarter of the roasted butternut squash for lunch on day 8.

Butternut Squash, Quinoa & Chicken Pot

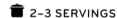 **2–3 SERVINGS**

500g (1lb 2oz) peeled butternut squash, diced
2 tablespoons olive oil
2 teaspoons ground cumin*
½ onion, chopped
140g (5oz) skinless chicken breast, diced (optional)
300g (10½oz) canned chopped tomatoes
300ml (½ pint) water
200g (7oz) canned chickpeas, rinsed and drained (optional)
finely grated zest of 1 lemon
juice of ½ lemon
8 cherry tomatoes, halved
80g (3oz) dry quinoa
sea salt flakes and pepper
handful of chopped fresh coriander, to serve

Preheat the oven to 200°C (400°F), Gas Mark 6. Place the butternut squash in a roasting tin, lightly coat it with oil, season to taste and bake for 30 minutes, or until tender. Set aside one-quarter of the squash and store in an airtight container in the refrigerator for use later on in the week.

Heat the remaining oil in a large casserole over a low heat, add the cumin and onion and cook gently for about 5 minutes until softened.

Add the chicken, if using, and fry gently for a further 5–10 minutes until golden.

Add the canned tomatoes and measured water, cover and simmer gently for 20–30 minutes until the chicken is cooked through and the sauce has thickened.

Add the cooked butternut squash, chickpeas, if using, lemon zest and juice, cherry tomatoes and quinoa. Season to taste, cover and simmer for a further 10 minutes. Garnish with coriander before serving. Store the leftovers in an airtight container in the refrigerator overnight.

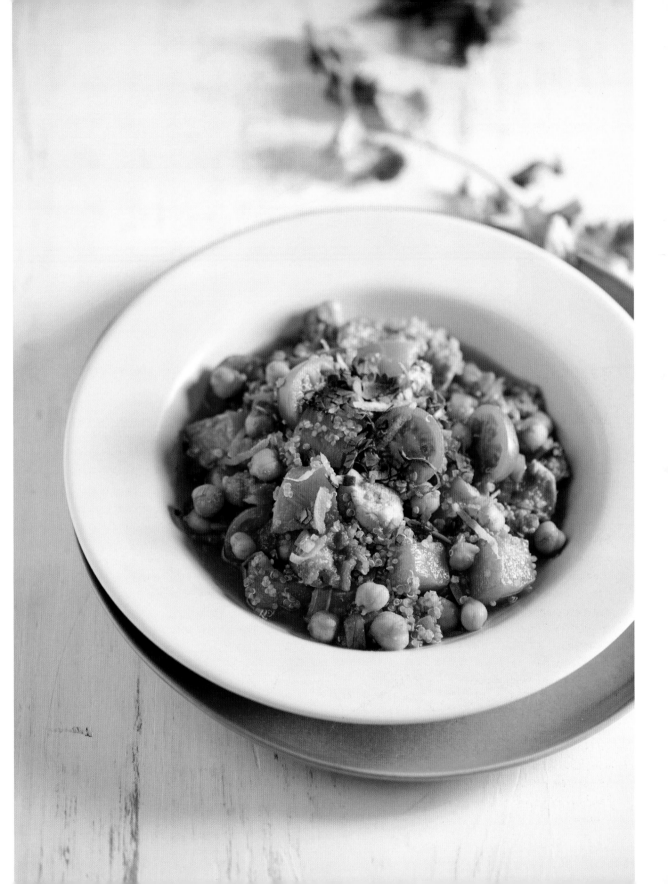

Warming Broth
with Vegetables, Noodles & Miso

1 SERVING

1 portion of Warming Broth (*see*
    page 61)
80g (3oz) pak choi, bean sprouts or
    broccoli (or a mixture)
40g (1½oz) rice noodles

OPTIONAL EXTRAS:
100g (3½oz) fish, tofu or tempeh
1–2 teaspoons miso paste
toasted seeds

Place the broth in a large saucepan over a medium heat and bring
to the boil. Add the vegetables and cook until the vegetables are just
tender, about 5–10 minutes.

Add the rice noodles and cook for another 2–3 minutes until softened.
If using fish, tofu or tempeh, add it to the soup with the noodles.

If using them, stir in the miso paste, or sprinkle with toasted seeds,
just before serving.

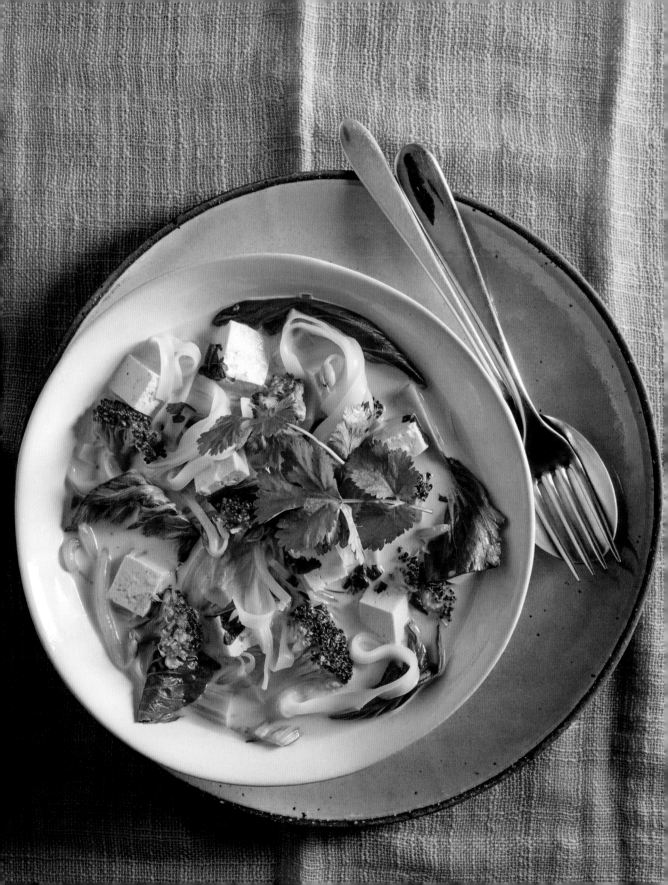

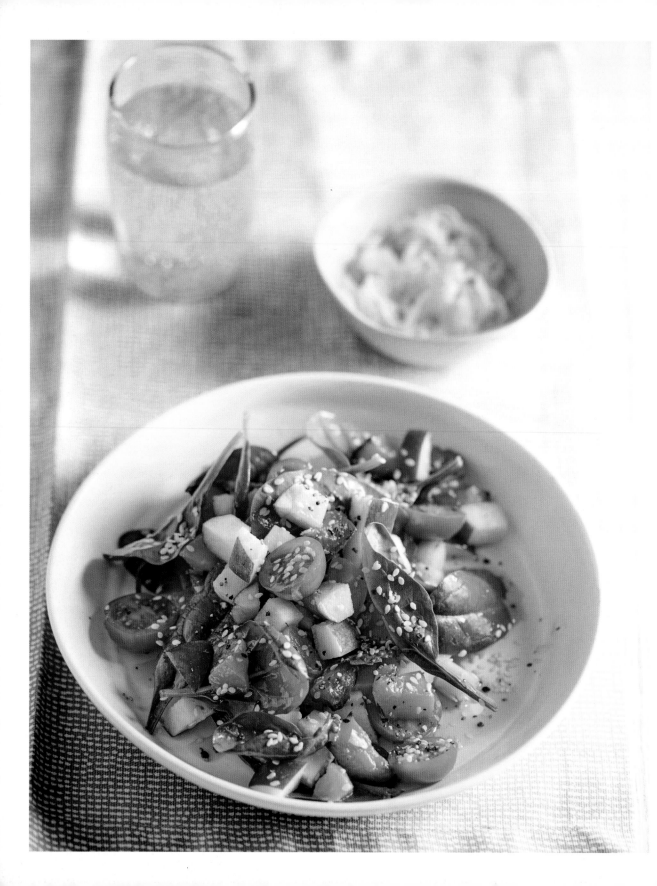

Butternut squash is rich in fibre, which will keep you full for longer, and also contains vitamin A and beta-carotene to support your gut lining. To increase the gut benefits, mix a tablespoon of sauerkraut or kimchi into this salad. Because these fermented vegetables have quite a strong taste, you may prefer to start with them on the side if you're not used to them.

Butternut Squash Salad

1 SERVING

butternut squash leftover from
    dinner on day 6 (*see* page 72)
1 handful of spinach
6 cherry tomatoes, halved
1½ teaspoons sesame seeds
1 apple, cored and diced (skin-on)
2 teaspoons extra virgin olive oil
juice of ½ lemon
sea salt flakes and pepper
1 tablespoon sauerkraut or kimchi,
    to serve (optional)

Place all the ingredients in a bowl and toss well to mix. Season to taste. If using, mix in the sauerkraut or kimchi, or serve on the side.

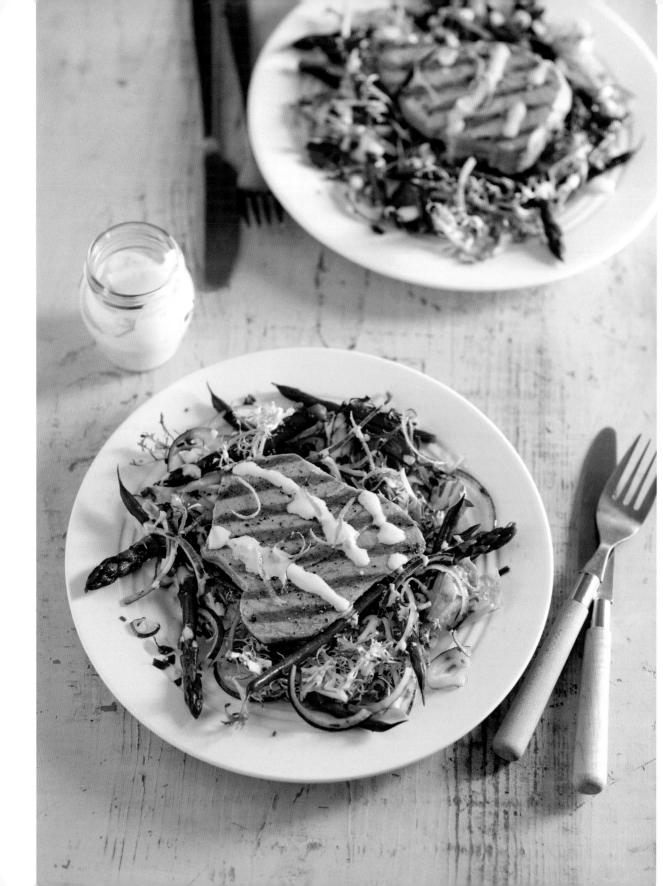

Tuna contains high amounts of niacin (vitamin B3) which is essential for optimum carbohydrate metabolism. The kefir in the dressing offers valuable probiotics to rebalance your gut bacteria levels. If you find raw onion hard to digest, sweat it lightly in a pan before adding to the salad. Don't forget to save half the finished dish for lunch tomorrow.

Pan-fried Tuna, Tofu or Eggs with Green Beans & Lemony Kefir Dressing

DAYS 8 & 9

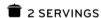 **2 SERVINGS**

18 green beans
6 asparagus spears, woody ends
   snapped off
½ red onion, sliced*
2 parsley sprigs, chopped
1 tablespoon olive oil, plus extra
   for greasing
50ml (2fl oz) kefir
finely grated zest of 1 lemon
2 handfuls of salad leaves
sea salt flakes and pepper

PROTEIN OF YOUR CHOICE, ABOUT 100G (3½OZ):
2 fresh tuna steaks
1 block of tofu
or 4 eggs

If using tofu, drain off the liquid, wrap the tofu in kitchen paper and place between 2 plates. Put a weight on top and leave for 30 minutes to remove some of the moisture.

If using eggs, boil the eggs in a saucepan of salted water for 4–5 minutes until just hard, then plunge into cold water to cool. Peel off the shells and cut the eggs in half.

Cook the green beans and asparagus in a saucepan of lightly salted water for about 3–5 minutes (depending on their size) until tender, then drain and place them in a bowl.

Add the red onion, parsley and oil, season to taste and mix well.

Place the kefir in a small bowl with the lemon zest. Season lightly and mix well.

Heat a lightly greased frying pan over a high heat and sear the tuna or tofu, if using, until golden and cooked to your liking.

Arrange the salad leaves on 2 plates and top with the green bean salad. Place the tuna, tofu or eggs on top and drizzle with the lemony kefir dressing. Cover and set aside one portion in the refrigerator for tomorrow, then tuck in.

Chickpeas are a valuable source of plant proteins and are rich in iron and manganese, which support energy production. Try to find organic chickpeas if you can. Freeze half of the finished dish for an instant dinner later in the plan.

Spanish Style Chickpeas

🍲 2 SERVINGS

225g (8oz) dried chickpeas, soaked overnight in cold water, or 800g (1lb 12oz) canned chickpeas, rinsed and drained
1–2 tablespoons olive oil
1 red pepper, cored, deseeded and chopped
450g (1lb) fresh tomatoes, chopped, or 400g (14oz) canned chopped tomatoes
½ teaspoon paprika
pinch of ground ginger*
pinch of ground coriander
pinch of ground nutmeg
pinch of black pepper
175g (6oz) dry quinoa, cooked according to packet instructions
sea salt flakes and pepper, to taste
2 handfuls of rocket and/or spinach leaves, to serve

If using dried chickpeas, rinse them well, place in a large saucepan and cover with water. Add 1 tablespoon of the olive oil, place over a high heat and bring to the boil. Reduce the heat and simmer for about 1½ hours or until the chickpeas are tender. Drain and set aside.

Heat 1 tablespoon of oil in a large frying pan and add the red pepper, tomatoes and spices. Cook the vegetables for about 10 minutes, stirring from time to time, until tender. Add the chickpeas and stir well to combine.

Serve half the chickpeas with the quinoa and rocket or spinach. Freeze the remainder in an airtight container for later.

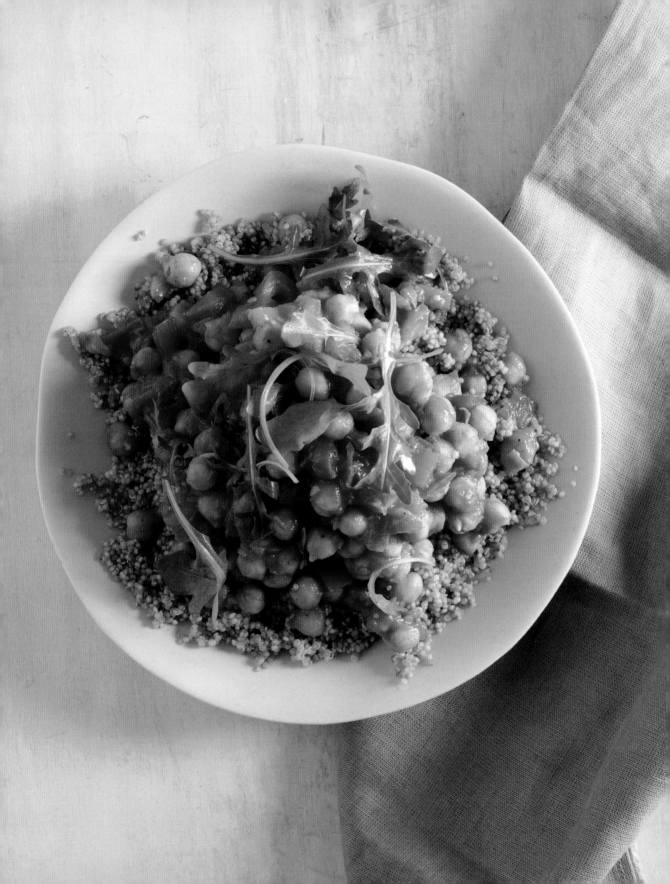

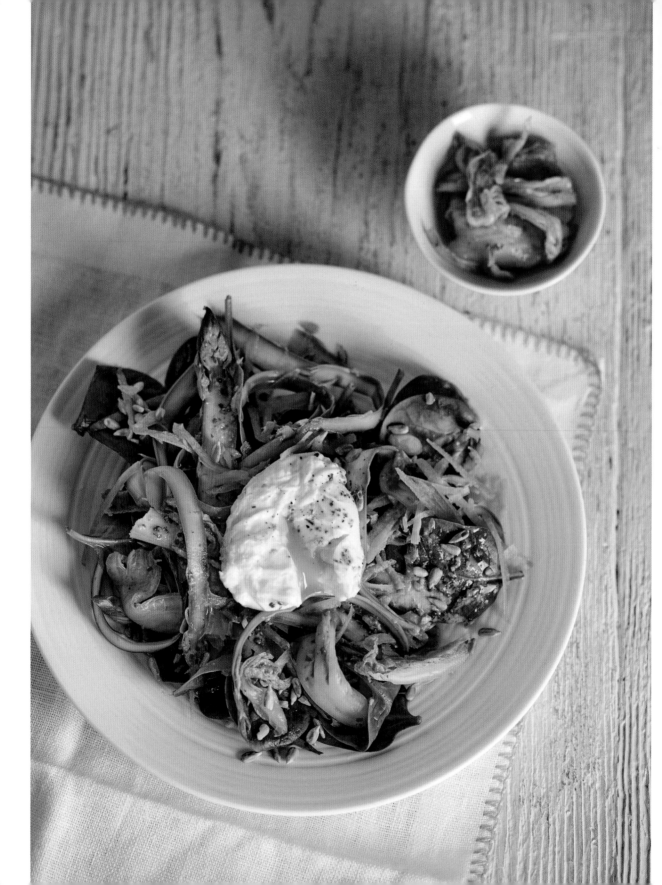

Asparagus, especially raw, is so good for your gut. It contains a special type of fibre called inulin, which is a prebiotic food for your microbiota. If you don't fancy eating it raw, you can lightly steam it. Boost bacteria levels by adding a spoonful of fermented pickles on the side.

Shaved Asparagus Salad

1 SERVING

1 bunch of asparagus
1 large handful of baby spinach
1 large carrot, grated
2 spring onions, chopped
1 tablespoon extra virgin olive oil
juice of ½ lemon
1 teaspoon wholegrain mustard
small handful of sunflower seeds
sea salt flakes and pepper, to taste

OPTIONAL EXTRAS:
1 poached egg
1 tablespoon sauerkraut or kimchi

Break off the woody ends of the asparagus and discard them, or save them to add to vegetable stock. 'Shave' the asparagus spears thinly using a vegetable peeler, or slice very thinly with a sharp knife and place in a large bowl.

Add the spinach, carrot and spring onions and toss together well.

Place the olive oil, lemon juice and mustard in a small bowl and whisk together, then drizzle over the salad.

Mix well and sprinkle with the sunflower seeds. Serve with a poached egg, and sauerkraut or kimchi on the side, if you like.

This Asian-inspired dish is super-delicious. The ginger will help stabilize blood sugar and is an anti-inflammatory. We've added a cup of miso soup on the side to boost the probiotic benefits. You can drink it before or alongside this meal. Save half the stir-fry for lunch tomorrow.

Super Stir-fry with Miso Soup

DAYS 10 & 11

2 SERVINGS

140g (5oz) rice noodles
1 tablespoon olive oil
4 garlic* cloves, chopped
4cm (1½ inches) fresh root ginger*,
    cut into matchsticks
1 head of broccoli, chopped
2 pak choi, chopped
2 handfuls of thinly sliced
    mushrooms
juice of 1 lime
4 tablespoons tamari soy sauce
1 handful of chopped fresh
    coriander
4 spring onions, sliced
50–70g (1¾–2½oz) mixed nuts and
    seeds, lightly toasted

YOUR CHOICE OF PROTEIN, ABOUT 100G (3½OZ):
½ block of tempeh, diced
1 lean chicken breast, diced
or 1 salmon fillet, diced

MISO SOUP:
1 teaspoon miso paste
200ml (7fl oz) boiling water

Soak the rice noodles in a bowl of hot water for 15 minutes until softened.

While the noodles are soaking, heat the olive oil in a wok until hot and add the garlic and ginger. Stir-fry for 30 seconds.

Add the broccoli and pak choi and stir-fry for 2 minutes.

Add the mushrooms and your choice of protein to the wok and continue to stir-fry until cooked through.

Add the lime juice and tamari, then drain the noodles and add them to the wok with the chopped coriander.

Toss well together and sprinkle with the spring onions and toasted nuts and seeds. Set aside half the stir-fry and store in an airtight container in the refrigerator overnight.

Make the miso soup by dissolving the paste in the measured boiling water and serve in a mug or bowl alongside your meal.

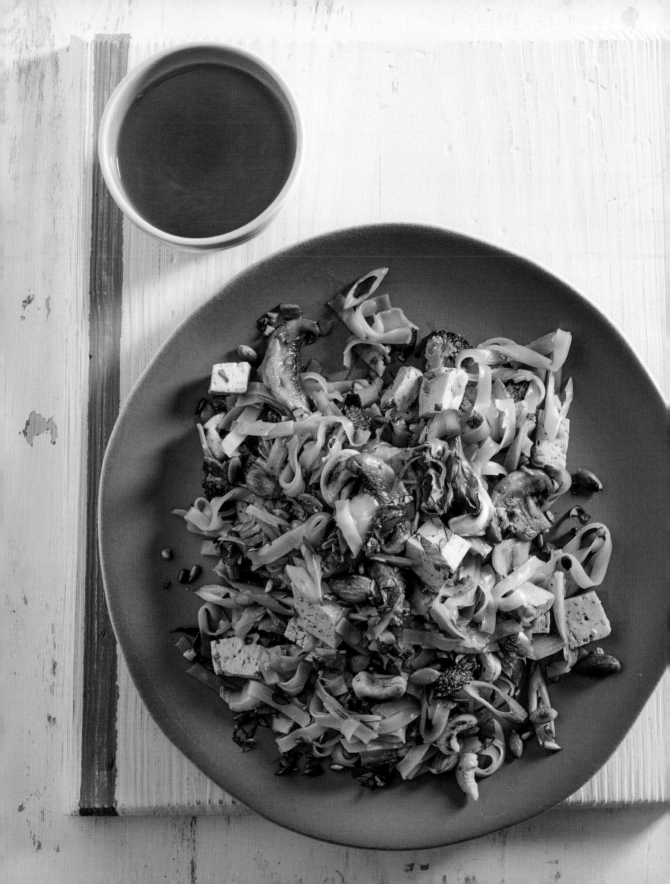

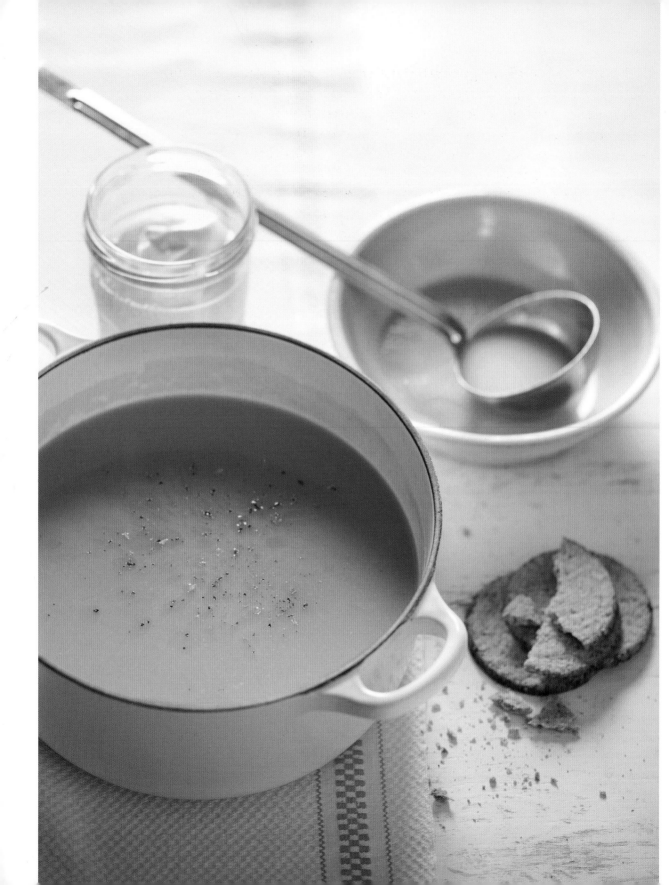

This great low-calorie energy booster is full of beta-carotene and can be made using pumpkin or butternut squash. Simple and nourishing, it's ideal when you need warming from the inside. Jerusalem artichokes are not related to the more familiar globe artichokes, rather, they look like nobbly ginger root and are super prebiotics to keep your friendly bacteria well fed and happy. They're in season from November to March so don't worry if you can't get them, just leave them out or replace with 2 small white potatoes. This recipe will make four portions. Enjoy one tonight, save one for lunch tomorrow, and freeze the remaining portions for a simple lunch or dinner when you don't have time to cook.

Pumpkin Soup with
Jerusalem Artichokes

DAYS 11 & 12

4 SERVINGS

1 tablespoon olive oil

1 onion, chopped

4 garlic* cloves, chopped

2 teaspoons grated fresh root
  ginger* (optional)

350g (12oz) peeled pumpkin or
  butternut squash, diced

300g (10½oz) Jerusalem
  artichokes, diced

about 1.2 litres (2 pints) water

pepper

TO SERVE:

soya milk, crème fraîche or natural
  yogurt (optional)

gluten-free oatcakes

Heat the oil in a large saucepan over a medium heat and add the onion, garlic and ginger, if using. Cook for about 5 minutes until softened, then add the vegetables and stir well.

Add the measured water and bring to the boil, then cover, reduce the heat and simmer for about 20 minutes until the vegetables are tender.

Alternatively, if making in advance you can slow-cook the soup by bringing it to the boil, and then turning off the heat and leaving it for at least 1 hour.

Season to taste, then blend until smooth using a hand-held blender or a food processor.

Pour one-quarter of the soup into a bowl and stir in a little soya milk, crème fraîche or natural yogurt, if using, to make it creamier. Serve with gluten-free oatcakes.

Store another portion in an airtight container in the refrigerator overnight, then freeze the remaining two portions for later.

The latest spice to be hailed a superfood, turmeric contains a compound called curcumin, which has been shown to reduce inflammation. Adding a spoon of sauerkraut or kimchi on the side helps to increase the levels and diversity of bacteria living in your gut.

Green Salad with Turmeric Dressing

1 SERVING

1 head of Romaine or lettuce, sliced
1 large handful of spinach
½ cucumber, diced
1–2 tablespoons sunflower and/or
  poppy seeds
1 tablespoon sauerkraut or kimchi,
  to serve (optional)

YOUR CHOICE OF PROTEIN, ABOUT 100G (3½OZ):
1 cooked mackerel fillet
1 cooked chicken breast
or 2 soft-boiled eggs

DRESSING:
3 tablespoons tahini
4 tablespoons lemon juice
1 tablespoon olive oil
1 teaspoon ground turmeric
1 garlic* clove, grated
1 teaspoon ground coriander
½ teaspoon dried basil
¼–½ teaspoon cayenne pepper*
¼ teaspoon ground ginger*
sea salt flakes and pepper

Place all the dressing ingredients in a small blender, season to taste and blend briefly until well mixed.

Place all the salad ingredients in a bowl and drizzle with dressing, to taste. Serve the salad with your choice of protein, and a spoonful of sauerkraut or kimchi on the side, if using.

Any leftover dressing can be stored in an airtight container in the refrigerator for up to 3 days.

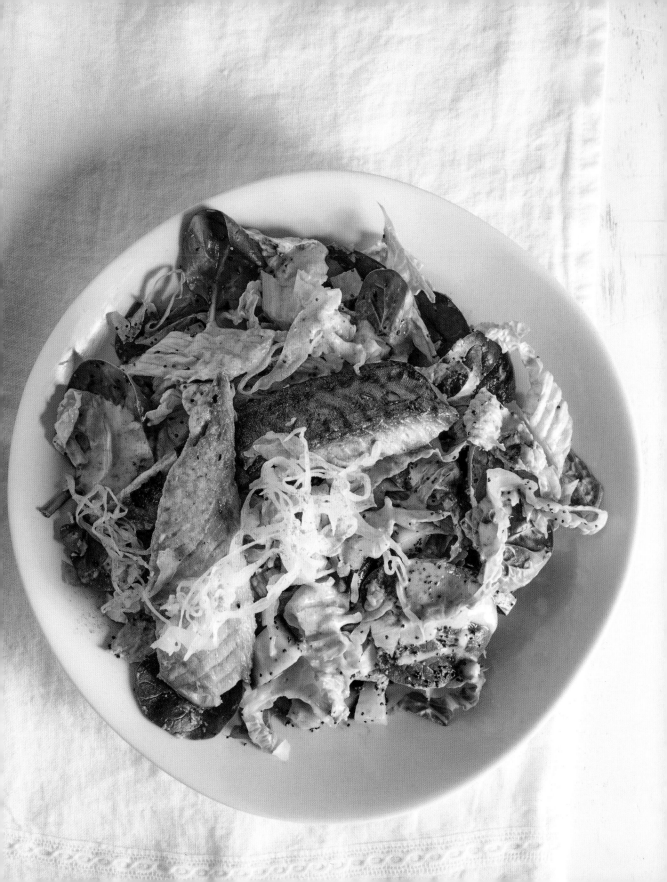

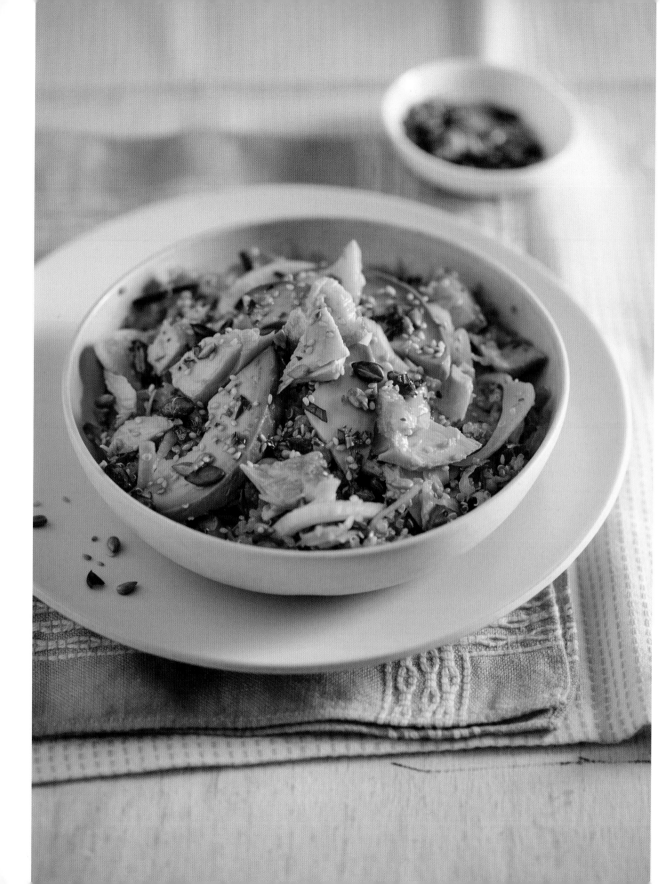

Fennel is a wonderful prebiotic food, helping to feed the good bacteria you've been restoring in your gut. If you've run out of quinoa or fancy a change, brown basmati rice, spelt or bulgur wheat can be used instead. You only need to peel the carrots before grating if they are not organic. The quinoa and seeds provide protein in this dish, but you can add additional protein if you wish, such as chicken, turkey, fish or tempeh. This recipe makes 2 portions, so save half for lunch tomorrow.

Warm Grain & Fennel Salad

DAYS 13 & 14

2 SERVINGS

80g (3oz) dry quinoa or other grain, cooked according to packet instructions
2 carrots, grated
1 fennel bulb, thinly sliced
1 cucumber, grated or finely sliced
1 avocado, sliced
2 tablespoons lightly toasted seeds (pumpkin, sesame, sunflower)
1 tablespoon sauerkraut or kimchi, to serve (optional)

YOUR CHOICE OF EXTRA PROTEIN, ABOUT 75–100G (2½–3½OZ):
cooked fish or tempeh
cooked chicken
or cooked turkey

DRESSING:
2 tablespoons extra virgin olive oil
2 tablespoons lemon juice
1 tablespoon finely chopped basil
sea salt flakes and pepper

Place the quinoa in a large bowl, then mix in the carrots, fennel and cucumber.

Place the dressing ingredients in a small bowl and whisk to combine, adding 2–4 tablespoons water to thin, if necessary. Pour over the salad and toss well, then top with the sliced avocado and sprinkle with the seeds.

Serve half the salad with your choice of extra protein and pickles on the side, if you like.

Set the remaining salad aside and store in an airtight container in the refrigerator overnight.

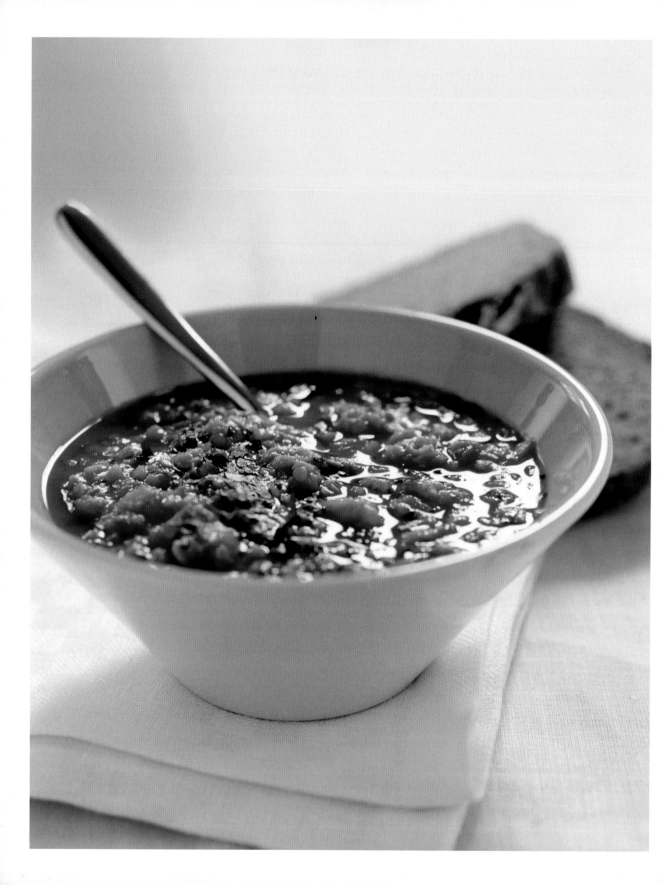

Lentils are very filling so are excellent in the fight against cravings and low blood sugar. They are also full of cholesterol-lowering fibre. Red split lentils cook quickly and do not require soaking, so they are perfect for a quick and simple supper. This recipe makes four portions: enjoy one today, one tomorrow, and freeze the remaining portions for Phase 3. You can throw any green vegetables into this soup when you reheat the leftovers.

Lebanese Lentil Soup

DAYS 14 & 15

🥘 4 SERVINGS

1 tablespoon olive oil

1 onion, finely chopped

4 garlic* cloves, crushed to a paste
   with a pinch of salt

1 teaspoon ground turmeric

1½ teaspoons ground cumin*

2 litres (3½ pints) water

400g (14oz) dried red split lentils,
   rinsed

1 bunch of Swiss chard or spinach,
   torn

juice of 2 large lemons

pepper

chopped coriander, to serve

Heat the oil in a large saucepan over a medium heat and cook the onion, garlic and spices for 5–10 minutes, or until soft.

Add the measured water and lentils and bring to the boil. Reduce the heat and simmer for about 20 minutes until the lentils are starting to fall apart, adding the chard or spinach for the final 5 minutes of cooking time.

Remove from the heat, stir in the lemon juice and season generously with black pepper. Pour one-quarter of the soup into a bowl and serve garnished with chopped coriander.

Store another portion in an airtight container in the refrigerator overnight, then freeze the other two portions for later.

This salad combines prebiotic-rich sprouted seeds with kale, which is rich in magnesium, iron and B vitamins, to keep your digestion and energy levels – and you – running smoothly. Nutrient-packed sprouted seeds, such as alfalfa, clover, radish or broccoli, are available in most large supermarkets or health-food shops in the fresh salad ingredients aisle.

Kale & Avocado Salad

DAY 16

1 SERVING

1 large handful of kale, chopped, tough stalks removed
60g (2¼oz) dry quinoa or brown basmati rice, cooked according to packet instructions
1 small carrot, grated
1 handful of sprouted seeds
1 handful of fresh herbs, such as basil, parsley or coriander
½ avocado, sliced
1 handful of cashew nuts or almonds, lightly toasted

DRESSING:
2–3 teaspoons miso paste
1 tablespoon extra virgin olive oil
juice of ½ lemon

Lightly cook the kale in a steamer set over a saucepan of gently simmering water until tender.

Drain and place in a large bowl with the cooked quinoa or rice, the carrot, sprouted seeds and herbs.

Place the dressing ingredients in a small bowl and whisk together, thinning with a little water to get the desired consistency. Pour over the salad ingredients and toss well to mix. Serve the salad topped with the sliced avocado and toasted nuts.

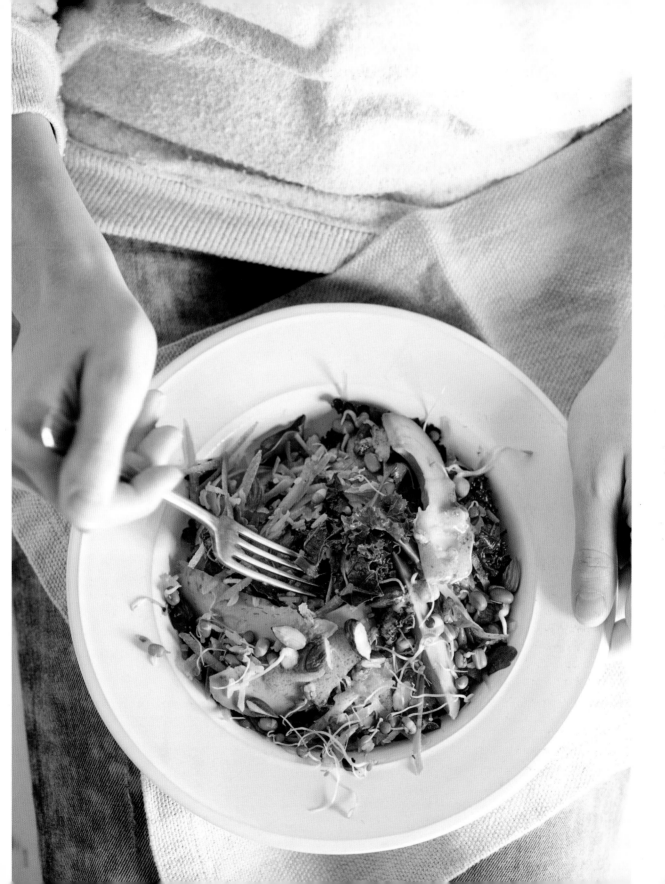

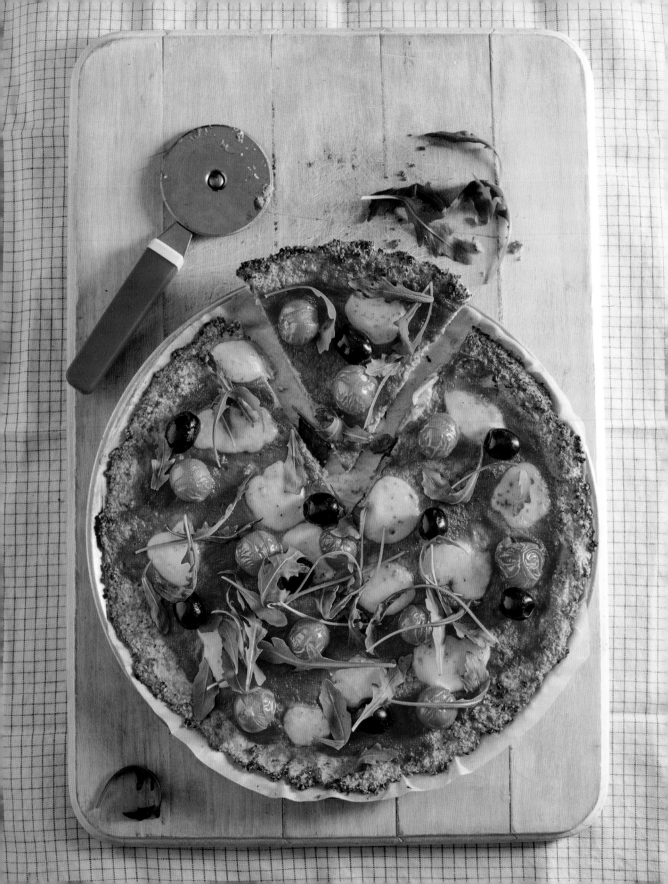

A low-carb alternative to a family favourite, this pizza is designed to boost your vegetable intake without boosting your waistline. It serves 2, so share with a friend.

Cauli-Pizza

2 SERVINGS

1 cauliflower, divided into florets
oil, for brushing
100g (3½oz) ground almonds
2 eggs, beaten
70g (2½oz) Parmesan cheese,
   grated
150ml (¼ pint) fresh tomato sauce
   or shop-bought passata
125g (4½oz) mozzarella, sliced, or
   6–8 mini balls
1 handful of pitted black olives
1 handful of cherry tomatoes
rocket or basil leaves, to serve

Place the cauliflower florets in a food processor and blend until finely chopped, like rice. You may have to do this in several batches.

Place the chopped cauliflower in a dry frying pan and cook for about 10 minutes, stirring occasionally, to evaporate all of the moisture. Alternatively, put it into a microwaveable bowl, cover with clingfilm and cook in the microwave for 5–6 minutes.

Preheat the oven to 180°C (350°F), Gas Mark 4. Line a large baking sheet with baking paper and brush with oil.

Spread the cauliflower out on a clean tea towel and leave to cool, so the moisture can evaporate. Once cool, pick up the corners of the tea towel and squeeze any remaining liquid out of the cauliflower.

Transfer to a mixing bowl and stir in the ground almonds, eggs and grated Parmesan.

Tip the cauliflower mixture into the centre of the prepared baking sheet and spread it out into a round, about 1cm (½ inch) thick in the middle and thicker at the edges. Bake for 15–20 minutes until just turning golden.

Spread the pizza base evenly with the fresh tomato sauce and arrange the mozzarella, olives and tomatoes on top. Bake for a further 8–10 minutes until the topping is bubbling. Serve topped with as much rocket or basil as you like.

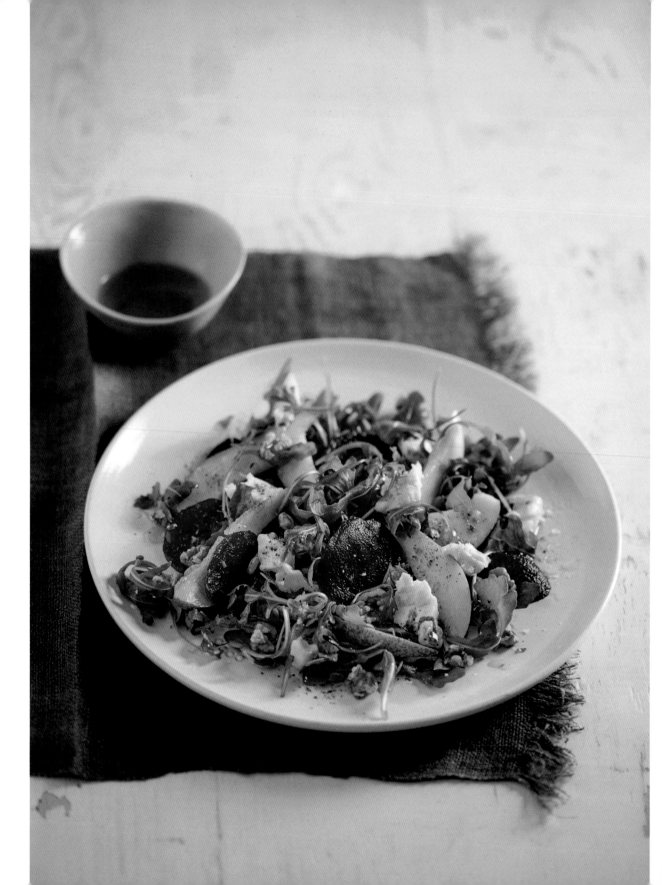

Rocket is a great peppery food that helps to stimulate your digestive juices, while beetroot is rich in heart-healthy antioxidants. Buy precooked beetroot, or roast whole raw beetroot in the oven for 30–40 minutes until tender, then peel it. We've added Gorgonzola to this recipe because it's a fermented cheese which contains abundant numbers and varieties of gut-friendly bacteria. However, swap for another cheese such as goats' cheese if you don't like the taste. You could also use Roquefort or another blue cheese if you prefer. Look for unpasteurized cheeses if possible.

Rocket, Walnut & Beetroot Salad with Gorgonzola

DAY 17

1 SERVING

60g (2¼oz) rocket
1 large, cooked beetroot, sliced
1 large, firm pear, cored and sliced
30g (1oz) walnuts, broken into
   pieces
40g (1½oz) Gorgonzola cheese

DRESSING:

1–2 tablespoons extra virgin
   olive oil
1 tablespoon lime or lemon juice
sea salt flakes and pepper

Place the dressing ingredients in a small bowl, season to taste and whisk well.

Arrange the rocket on a plate, add the sliced beetroot and pears, top with the walnut pieces and crumble over the Gorgonzola. Pour over the dressing and enjoy.

Asparagus contains a number of anti-inflammatory nutrients as well as having prebiotic properties, making it particularly supportive for the gut. Add kefir for a probiotic boost. Save a portion for lunch tomorrow.

Asparagus Soup

2 SERVINGS

1 tablespoon olive oil
1 garlic clove, chopped
250g (9oz) asparagus spears, plus
  an extra handful to garnish,
  woody stems snapped off, and
  roughly chopped
500ml (18fl oz) hot vegetable stock
  (*see* page 60)
sea salt flakes and pepper
kefir, to serve (optional)
toasted rye bread, to serve

Heat the oil in a large saucepan over a low heat, add the garlic and cook until soft, about a minute. Add the asparagus and a pinch of sea salt and cook for a further couple of minutes.

Add the stock and bring to the boil. Reduce the heat and simmer for about 5 minutes until the asparagus is tender. Reserve a handful of asparagus spears to garnish. Blend the remaining asparagus soup until smooth using a hand-held blender or a food processor. Season to taste.

Pour half of the soup into a bowl and garnish with half of the reserved asparagus spears. If using, drizzle over some kefir. Serve with a slice of toasted rye bread.

Set aside another portion and the remaining reserved spears and store in an airtight container in the refrigerator overnight.

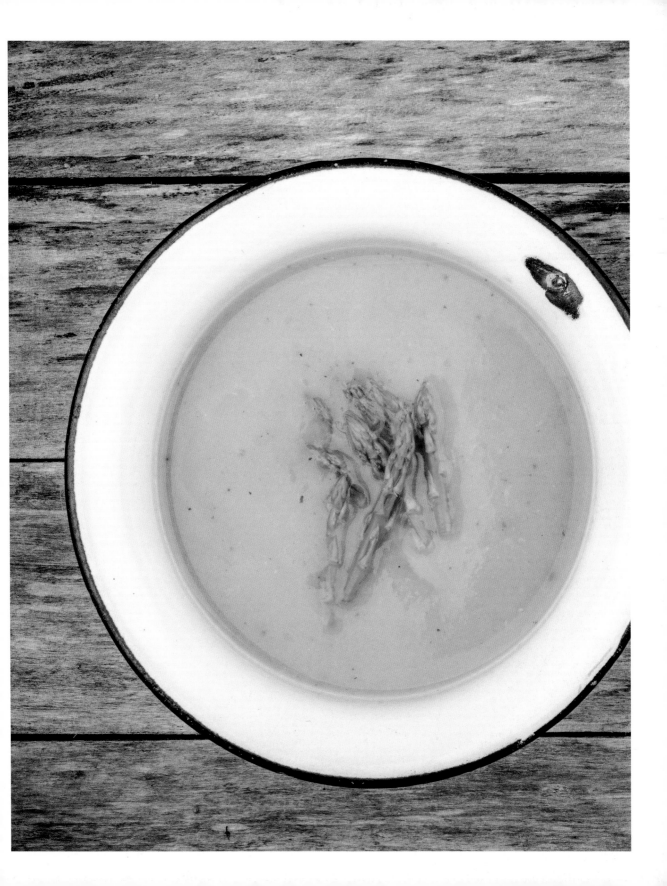

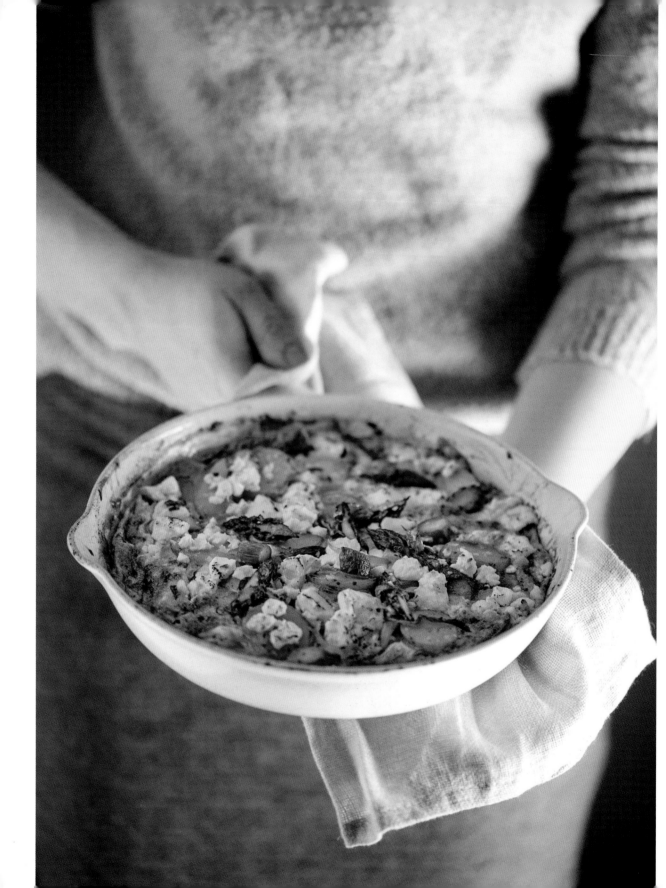

Eggs are an amazing source of vitamins, minerals, protein and the healthy low-density lipoprotein (LDL) cholesterol, which helps to support heart health. This frittata is a great way to get eggs into your diet and use up any vegetables you have in your refrigerator. Don't forget to save half the frittata for lunch tomorrow.

Vegetable Frittata

🍲 2 SERVINGS

1 tablespoon good-quality butter or
    coconut oil
½ onion, sliced
2 mushrooms, sliced
4 asparagus spears, woody ends
    snapped off, chopped
6 eggs
dash of almond milk
1 handful of fresh or dried herbs,
    such as basil or parsley, chopped
4 small Jerusalam artichokes or
    new potatoes, cooked and sliced
50g (1¾oz) feta cheese, crumbled
sea salt flakes and pepper
handful of rocket and/or
    watercress, to serve

Heat the butter or coconut oil in a frying pan over a medium heat, add the onion, mushrooms and asparagus and cook gently until softened.

Place the eggs in a bowl with the dash of almond milk and the herbs. Season to taste and whisk well.

Pour the egg mixture into the frying pan with the onion and mushrooms and cook over a low heat for 3–4 minutes until almost set. Sprinkle the potatoes and feta over the top then place under a preheated hot grill until the egg is cooked through.

Serve half the frittata immediately with rocket and/or watercress on the side. Set aside the remaining frittata and store in an airtight container in the refrigerator overnight.

Capsicum in chillies raises metabolism, don't use much if your tummy is sensitive. We've served this with brown rice for fibre, fresh spinach for an extra nutrient hit, and natural yogurt, which is rich in probiotics. If you feel bloated after eating rice, keep the portion small or swap it for grated, steamed cauliflower or a baked sweet potato, which may be easier to digest. Save half the Chilli for lunch tomorrow.

Chilli Con Carne

🍲 2 SERVINGS

1 tablespoon olive or coconut oil (optional)
1 onion, diced
1 red pepper, deseeded and diced
2 garlic* cloves, crushed
½–1 teaspoon mild chilli powder*
2 teaspoons paprika*
1 teaspoon ground cumin*
250ml (9fl oz) beef or vegetable stock (*see page 60*)
400g (14oz) canned chopped tomatoes
1 teaspoon tomato purée
small bunch of fresh coriander, chopped

YOUR CHOICE OF PROTEIN:

250g (9oz) good-quality minced steak
250g (9oz) good-quality minced turkey
400g (14oz) canned mixed beans, rinsed and drained
or 200g (7oz) Quorn mince

TO SERVE:

50–70g (1¾–2½oz) dried brown rice, per serving
handful of spinach, chopped
natural yogurt
sea salt flakes and pepper

Rinse the rice in cold water and drain. Place in a saucepan with about 400ml (14fl oz) of cold water, making sure the water covers the rice by at least 1–2cm (½–¾ inch). Bring to the boil, cover then reduce the heat and simmer for 20–25 minutes until the rice has absorbed the water and is cooked through.

Meanwhile, if using minced steak, place the onion and steak in a preheated frying pan over a medium heat and cook until browned. Do not add oil as there will be enough fat in the mince.

If using turkey, heat the oil in a frying pan over a medium heat and cook the onion and turkey until golden.

If using beans or Quorn, heat the oil in a frying pan over a medium heat and cook the onion until softened and golden.

Add the red pepper, garlic, chilli powder, paprika and cumin and fry gently for 1–2 minutes until fragrant.

Add the stock, tomatoes and tomato purée. If using mixed beans or Quorn as your protein, add that at this point too. Stir and allow to simmer for 10–15 minutes, or until the sauce is thick, then stir in the fresh coriander.

Serve half the Chilli with all the brown rice, the chopped spinach and a spoonful of yogurt. Set aside the remaining Chilli and store in an airtight container in the refrigerator overnight.

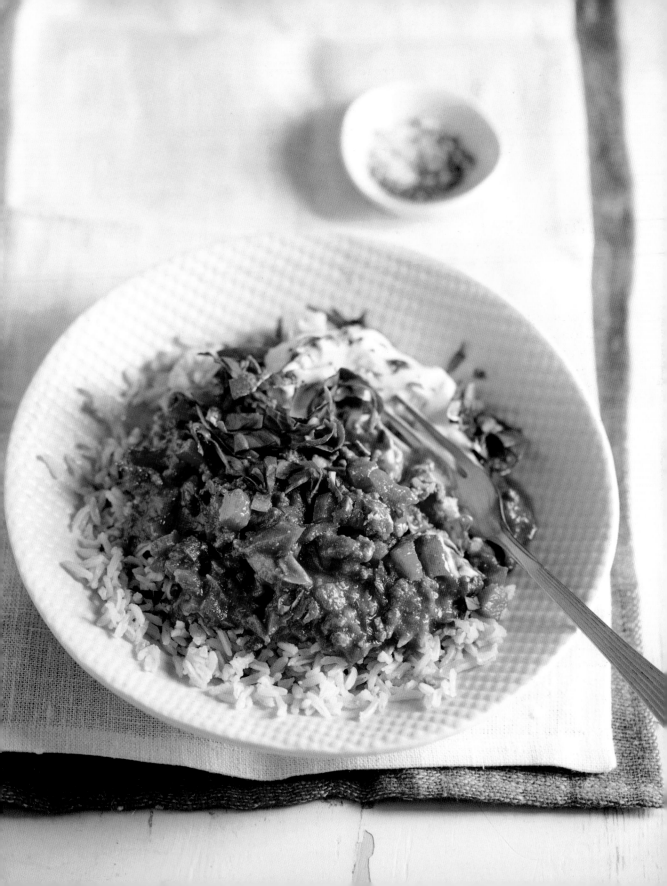

The sprouted seeds in this dish support digestive enzymes, while the prawns or chickpeas and quinoa provide protein to support overall health and wellbeing. You can switch the quinoa for brown basmati rice, spelt or buckwheat if you fancy a change. And feel free to add other vegetables if you have some that need using up. Save half the salad for lunch tomorrow.

Garlic Prawns with Quinoa Salad

DAYS 20 & 21

2 SERVINGS

120g (4½oz) dry quinoa or other grain

1 vegetable stock cube or 1 teaspoon powder

½ head of broccoli, grated or finely chopped

1 bunch of parsley, chopped

1 bunch of mint, chopped

4 tomatoes, diced

2 tablespoons extra virgin olive oil

2 tablespoons lemon juice

1 handful of sprouted seeds

FOR THE PRAWNS OR CHICKPEAS:

2 tablespoons extra virgin olive oil

2 garlic* cloves, crushed

1 handful of raw or cooked peeled prawns, or 100g (3½oz) canned chickpeas, rinsed and drained

Cook the quinoa or other grain according to the packet instructions, adding the vegetable stock cube or powder to the cooking water for extra flavour. Allow to cool to room temperature.

Place the quinoa in a bowl and add the broccoli, parsley, mint and tomatoes. Add the oil, lemon juice and sprouted seeds, then toss together well.

To cook the prawns or chickpeas, heat the oil in a frying pan over a high heat, add the garlic and cook briefly, then add the prawns or chickpeas and toss until cooked or warmed through.

Serve half the salad topped with all the prawns or chickpeas. Set aside the remaining salad and store in an airtight container in the refrigerator overnight.

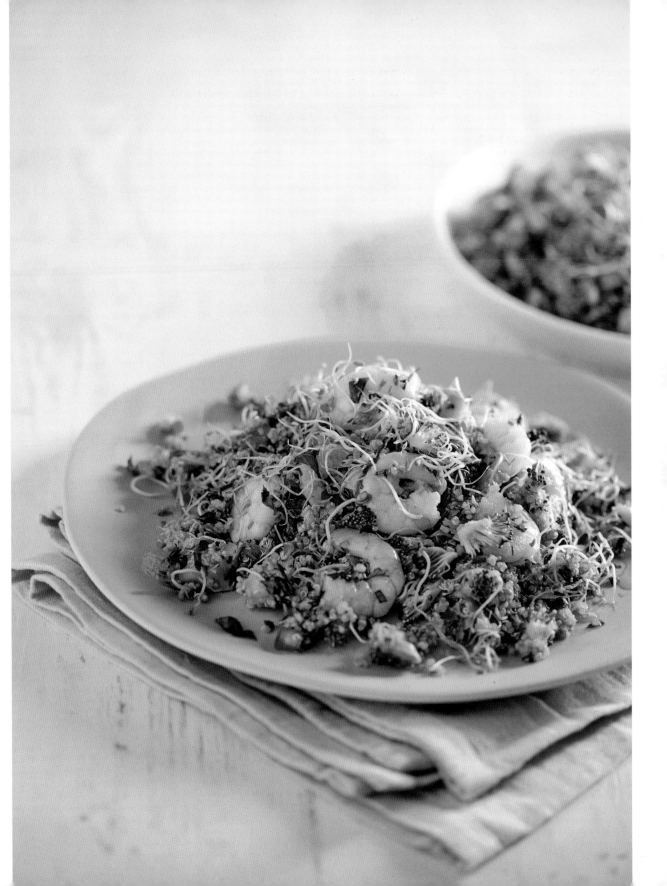

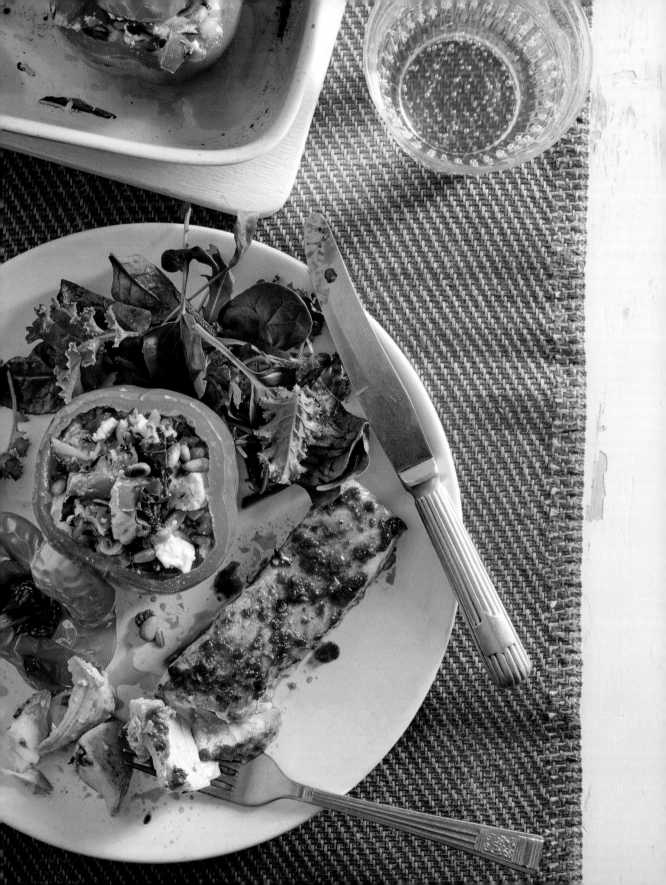

With its great balance of flavours and spices, this dish provides protein as well as vitamin C from the peppers, and antioxidants from the tomatoes.

Stuffed Peppers with Marinated Salmon or Chicken

DAY 21

2 SERVINGS

1 teaspoon harissa paste*
2 red peppers
1 tablespoon olive oil
1 tablespoon pine nuts
80g (3oz) feta cheese, crumbled
1 courgette, grated
1 tomato, diced
1 handful of chopped basil
sea salt flakes and pepper
green salad, to serve

YOUR CHOICE OF PROTEIN:
120g (4½oz) salmon fillet
120g (4½oz) chicken breast
or 200g (7oz) canned green lentils,
   rinsed and drained

Preheat the oven to 180°C (350°F), Gas Mark 4.

Rub the salmon fillet or chicken breast, if using, with the harissa paste and leave to marinate for 30 minutes. Transfer to an ovenproof dish, cover and bake the chicken for 25 minutes or the salmon for 15 minutes, until cooked through.

Slice the tops off the peppers and scoop out the seeds. Place in an ovenproof dish, drizzle with oil and bake for 10 minutes.

At the same time, spread the pine nuts on a baking sheet and bake for 5–7 minutes, stirring from time to time, until golden.

Place the pine nuts in a mixing bowl with the feta, courgette, tomato and basil. Season to taste and mix well. If using lentils, stir them into the vegetable mixture with the harissa.

Remove the peppers from the oven and stuff with the feta mixture. Take care – they'll be hot! Return the peppers to the oven and bake for 10–15 minutes.

Serve one stuffed pepper with your chicken or fish, if using, accompanied by a green salad.

Allow the other pepper to cool, then cover and store in the refrigerator overnight, and enjoy for lunch tomorrow with a mixed salad.

SNACKS

RAW ENERGY BALLS

PHASE 3 ONWARDS

Homemade energy balls make a tasty, healthy snack. These are packed with goodness and take only minutes to make. They can be stored in the refrigerator for up to 5 days, so make them on a Sunday for the week ahead. Each recipe makes about 10; a portion is 1 or 2 balls.

These are a source of B vitamins, which help your digestive system to derive fuel from your food, and are also rich in minerals such as beta-carotene and iron.

Superfood Balls

5–10 SERVINGS

50g (1¾oz) gluten-free oats
5 mint leaves
½ teaspoon ground ginger or grated fresh root ginger*
2 teaspoons spirulina
4 tablespoons flaxseeds
1 tablespoon manuka honey
5 dates, pitted
1 tablespoon sesame seeds, for coating

Place all the ingredients, except the sesame seeds, in a blender or food processor and blend to a dough.

Use a tablespoon to shape the dough into 10 balls. Spread the sesame seeds on a plate, then roll the balls in the seeds to coat. Store in an airtight container in the refrigerator for up to 1 week.

A deliciously good source of satisfying monounsaturated fats and soothing magnesium, a vital nutrient for good digestion.

Unsweetened coconut flakes are available in health-food shops. Peel the carrot before grating if it isn't organic.

Pecan Pie Balls

5–10 SERVINGS

100g (3½oz) pecan nuts
4 tablespoons gluten-free oats
½ teaspoon ground cinnamon
¼ teaspoon ground ginger*
¼ teaspoon ground cloves
¼ teaspoon grated nutmeg
4 dates, pitted
80g (3oz) dried apricots

FOR COATING:
1 tablespoon chia seeds
1 tablespoon flaxseeds

Place the pecan nuts in a dry frying pan over a medium heat for 2–3 minutes, stirring frequently, until lightly toasted.

Transfer the nuts to a blender or food processor and pulse until chopped. Add the oats and spices and pulse until combined. Add the fruits and blend to a dough.

Use a tablespoon to shape the dough into 10 balls. Spread the chia and flaxseeds on a plate, then roll the balls in the seeds to coat. Store in an airtight container in the refrigerator for up to 1 week.

Carrot Cake Balls

5–10 SERVINGS

180ml (6fl oz) water
60g (2¼oz) buckwheat
50g (1¾oz) oats
25g (1oz) unsweetened coconut flakes
1 carrot, grated
finely grated zest of 1 orange
1 teaspoon ground cinnamon
1 tablespoon raw honey
unsweetened desiccated coconut, for coating

Place the water in a saucepan and bring to the boil. Add the buckwheat, reduce the heat and simmer, covered, for about 10 minutes until all water has been absorbed and the buckwheat is tender. Leave to cool.

Place the oats in a blender or food processor and blend until fine. Add the coconut flakes and blend again until fine. Add the cooled buckwheat and the remaining ingredients, except the dessicated coconut, and mix to a dough.

Use a tablespoon to shape the dough into 10 balls. Spread the desiccated coconut on a plate, then roll the balls in the coconut to coat. Store in an airtight container in the refrigerator for up to 1 week.

These pack a punch of protein, making them a great post-workout option, with the added health benefits of tummy-friendly chia seeds and anti-inflammatory turmeric.

Coconut flour is available from good health-food shops and is created from the remnants from making coconut products.

Sweet 'n' Salty Cookie Dough Balls

10 SERVINGS

60g (2¼oz) ground almonds
65g (2½oz) unsweetened peanut butter
1 teaspoon ground cinnamon
2 tablespoons chia seeds
½ teaspoon ground turmeric
1 teaspoon extra virgin coconut oil

FOR COATING:
1 tablespoon organic raw cocoa powder
1 tablespoon toasted salted hemp seeds

Place all the ingredients in a blender or food processor and blend to a dough.

Use a tablespoon to shape the dough into 10 balls, then dust them with the cocoa powder. Spread the hemp seeds on a plate, then roll the balls in the seeds to coat. Store in an airtight container for up to 1 week.

Coconut Lime Pie Balls

5–10 SERVINGS

60g (2¼oz) almonds (blanched or skin-on)
60g (2¼oz) brazil nuts
½ teaspoon ground cardamom
15g (½oz) desiccated coconut, plus extra for coating
3 tablespoons coconut flour
finely grated zest and juice of 2 limes
8 dates, pitted
1 tablespoon manuka honey

Place the almonds, brazil nuts, cardamom, desiccated coconut and coconut flour in a blender or food processor and pulse until combined. Add the remaining ingredients and mix to a dough.

Use a tablespoon to shape the dough into 10 balls. Spread some more desiccated coconut on a plate, then roll the balls in the coconut to lightly coat. Store in an airtight container in the refrigerator for up to 1 week.

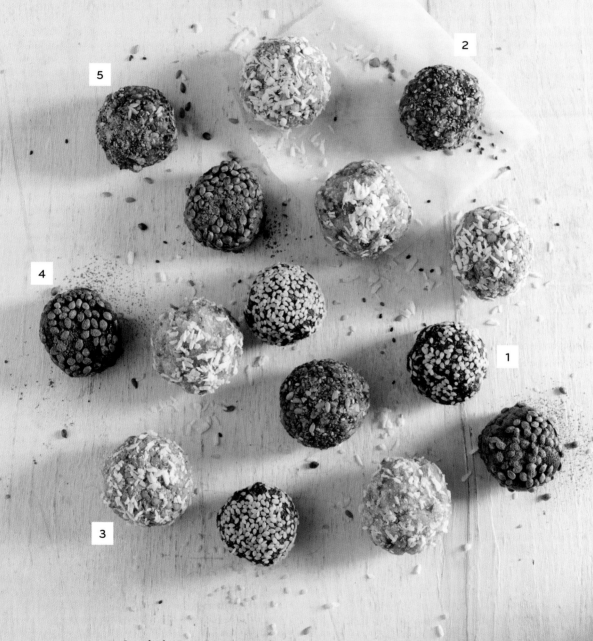

1. Superfood, 2. Pecan Pie, 3. Carrot Cake, 4. Sweet 'n' Salty Cookie Dough, 5. Coconut Lime Pie

Again these can be batch-cooked so you have a tasty, protein-packed snack when you need one through the week. One portion is 8–10 nuts.

Make a large batch and store in an airtight jar for when you fancy a sweet snack. Cinnamon tastes naturally sweet but doesn't spike your blood sugar. One portion is 1 tablespoon of seeds.

Savoury Nuts & Seeds

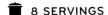 **8 SERVINGS**

60g (2¼oz) cashew nuts
60g (2¼oz) skin-on, unsalted almonds
60g (2¼oz) pumpkin or sunflower seeds
3 tablespoons tamari soy sauce

Preheat the oven to 180°C (350°F), Gas Mark 4.

Spread out the nuts and seeds on a baking sheet and bake for 10–15 minutes, stirring halfway through, until starting to brown.

As soon as you remove the baking sheet from the oven tip the nuts and seeds into a bowl, pour over the soy sauce and mix well to coat them all.

Allow to cool, then store in an airtight container.

Sweet Seeds

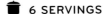 **6 SERVINGS**

2–3 teaspoons coconut oil
2 teaspoons ground cinnamon
6 tablespoons pumpkin and/or sunflower seeds

Preheat the oven to 150°C (300°F), Gas Mark 2.

Heat the coconut oil in a small saucepan over a low heat, then stir in the cinnamon and seeds until well coated.

Spread out on a baking sheet and bake for 20–30 minutes until crispy. Allow to cool, then store in an airtight container.

Almonds are proven to balance blood sugar levels after a meal, helping you avoid that dip which can make you feel sleepy after eating. This is also a great option if you fancy something sweeter without the sugar rush that comes with so many sweet treats. You can make your own almond butter using the recipe that follows or choose a shop-bought version with no added salt or sugar. Each serving is 2 tablespoons with 2–3 gluten-free oatcakes.

Cashew nuts are powerful antioxidants and studies show that a regular intake of nuts can lower your risk of heart disease. Each serving is 2 tablespoons with 2–3 gluten-free oatcakes.

Almond Butter

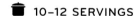 **10–12 SERVINGS**

250g (9oz) skin-on, unsalted almonds
apple slices or gluten-free oatcakes, to serve

Preheat the oven to 190°C (375°F), Gas Mark 5 and spread the almonds on a baking sheet.

Bake for 10–15 minutes until hot to the touch. Transfer the nuts to a blender or food processor and blend until smooth. It will take 15–20 minutes for the nuts to turn into butter, so be patient and stop the blender from time to time to scrape down the sides of the bowl. Store in the refrigerator for up to 3 days.

Cashew Nut Dip

 8–10 SERVINGS

250g (9oz) cashew nuts, soaked overnight
    in cold water and drained
4 tablespoons lemon juice
8 tablespoons olive oil
4 garlic* cloves, peeled
pinch of sea salt flakes
pinch of ground cumin*

TO GARNISH:
paprika*
chopped parsley

Place all the ingredients in a blender or food processor and blend to a smooth consistency, adding a little water to thin, if necessary. Serve garnished with a little paprika and chopped parsley. Store in the refrigerator for up to 3 days.

OPTION: After Phase 1, replace the cumin with ½ teaspoon of miso paste for an Asian flavour and a probiotic boost.

For those who struggle to digest chickpeas, this dip offers a simple, tasty alternative to traditional hummus. The coriander will add colour and support digestion. One portion is 2 tablespoons of hummus with 2–3 gluten-free oatcakes or some vegetable batons. Pictured opposite.

Hummus is high in fibre and protein, which will help you to feel full and keep your blood sugar levels balanced. Chickpeas are also rich in iron and manganese, which support energy production. Shop-bought hummus can be used, but choose an organic product with a short ingredients list. One portion is 2 tablespoons of hummus with 2–3 gluten-free oatcakes or some vegetable batons.

Courgette & Coriander Hummus

🍲 8–10 SERVINGS

300g (10½oz) courgettes, peeled and chopped
150–200ml (5–7fl oz) tahini
100ml (3½fl oz) cold-pressed extra virgin olive oil
3–4 garlic* cloves
1 handful of fresh coriander
1 teaspoon ground cumin*
2 teaspoons sea salt flakes
juice of 4 lemons
smoked paprika*, to garnish

Place all the ingredients in a blender or food processor and blend to a smooth consistency. Serve garnished with a little smoked paprika. Store in an airtight container in the refrigerator for up to 3 days.

Chickpea Hummus 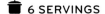 PHASE 2 ONWARDS

🍲 6 SERVINGS

400g (14oz) canned chickpeas, rinsed and drained
1 garlic clove
1 tablespoon tahini
pinch of sea salt flakes
juice of ½ lemon
3 tablespoons extra virgin olive oil
50ml (2fl oz) water

Place all the ingredients in a blender or food processor with the water and blend to a smooth consistency, adding a little more water to thin, if necessary. Store in an airtight container in the refrigerator for up to 3 days.

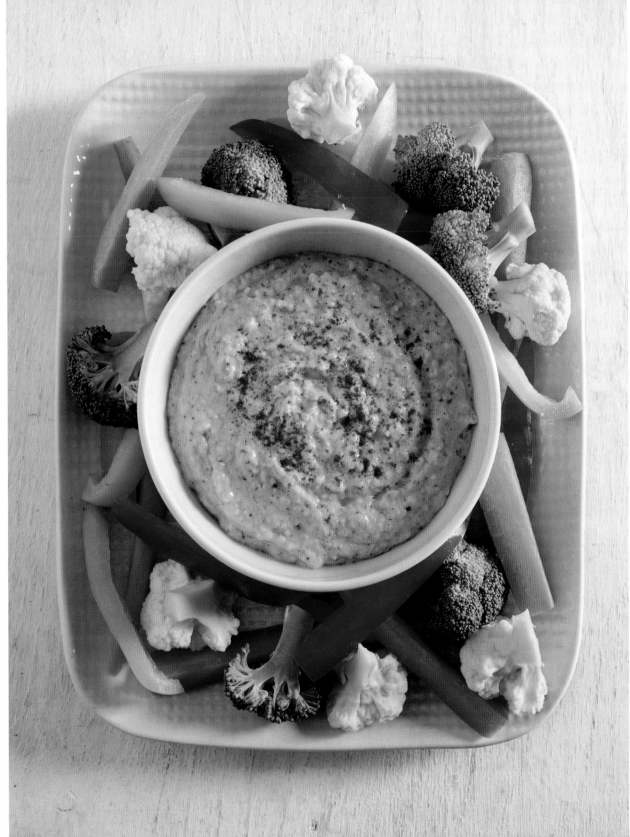

These brownies are sweetened with dates, which are lower on the glycaemic index (GI) than sugar, meaning they won't cause the same blood sugar spike. They're also high in fibre, potassium, iron and antioxidants. A portion is 1 brownie.

Raw Chocolate Brownies

PHASE 3 ONWARDS

10–12 SERVINGS

100g (3½oz) whole almonds with skin
250g (9oz) Medjool dates, pitted and chopped
2 tablespoons set raw honey
75g (2½oz) cocoa powder
½ teaspoon sea salt flakes
50g (1¾oz) pecan nuts, chopped

Place the almonds in a blender or food processor and blend until you have a coarse powder.

Add the dates, honey, cocoa and salt and mix until all the ingredients have combined into a sticky ball of dough.

Turn the dough out into a bowl, add the chopped pecan nuts and knead them in.

Line a 20-cm (8-inch) square baking tin with baking paper, turn the mixture into it and press it down with your fingers until it forms an even layer.

Chill for 30 minutes in the freezer (for faster chilling), then remove and score into 10–12 squares. Return to the freezer for a further 30 minutes until solid.

Store in an airtight container in the refrigerator for up to 1 week, or in the freezer for up to 4 weeks.

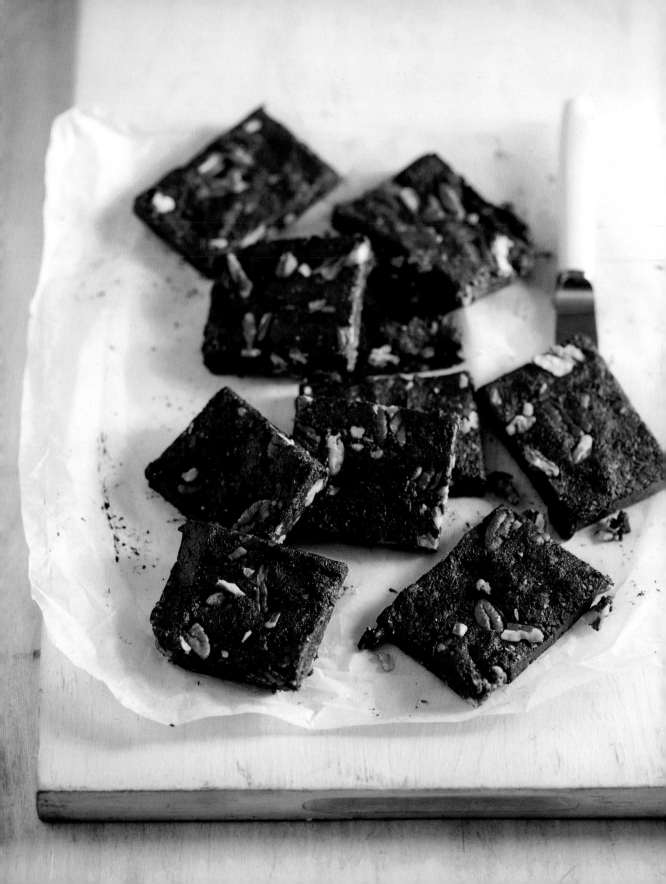

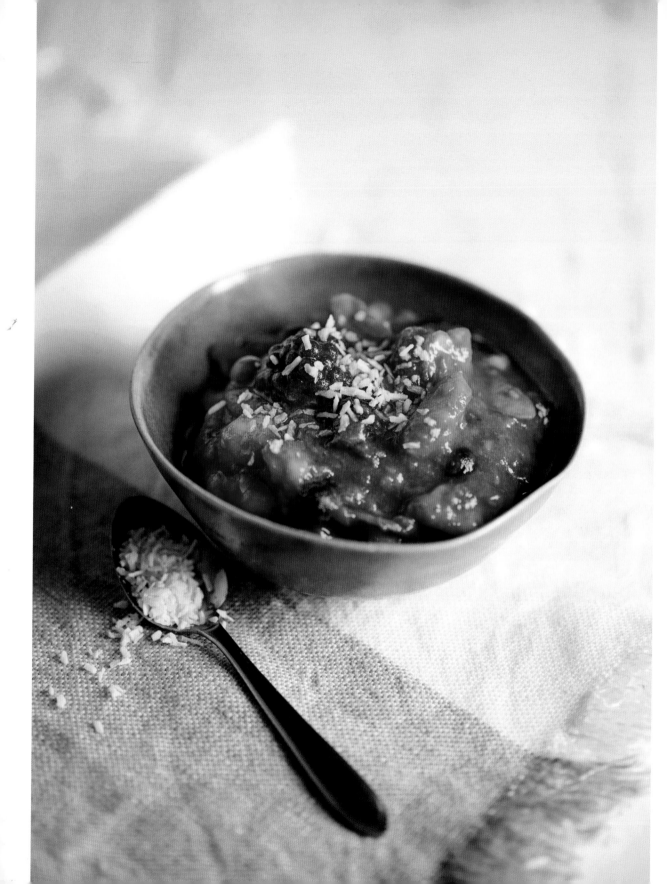

You can use any type of berry, or a mixture of more than one type, to make this tasty bake. All berries are extremely good for you and frozen berries are fine when fresh berries are not available. Pop into the oven when you're eating your main meal and they'll be perfectly cooked for pudding. Make a batch and save leftovers for a delicious compote.

Berry Banana Bake

PHASE 3 ONWARDS

1 SERVING

1 handful of fresh or frozen berries
½ banana, chopped
1 tablespoon flaked almonds

TO SERVE:
1 teaspoon desiccated coconut
natural yogurt or Greek yogurt, to
serve (optional)

Preheat the oven to 180°C (350°F), Gas Mark 4.

Place the berries, banana and almonds in a small ovenproof dish or ramekin and bake for 10–15 minutes, or until piping hot.

Serve with a sprinkling of desiccated coconut and a spoonful of yogurt, if liked.

This is a simple and nutritious pudding all the family will love. You can use other fruit to suit the season, like blackberries or rhubarb. You could even make a healthy topping with oats and ground almonds and pop it in the oven for a crumble. Children love this on top of porridge or cereal. Only add honey or another sweetener if you really need it.

Stewed Apples with Blueberries   PHASE 3 ONWARDS

4–6 SERVINGS

3–4 cooking apples, peeled, cored
   and chopped
1 teaspoon ground cinnamon
a drizzle of raw honey, maple syrup,
   agave syrup or other natural
   sweetener (optional)

TO SERVE:
natural yogurt or Greek yogurt
1 handful of blueberries

Place the apples in a saucepan over a low heat with the cinnamon and a dash of water and cook gently for 5–10 minutes until soft.

Taste and add a very small amount of your chosen sweetener, if liked.

Serve topped with yogurt and blueberries.

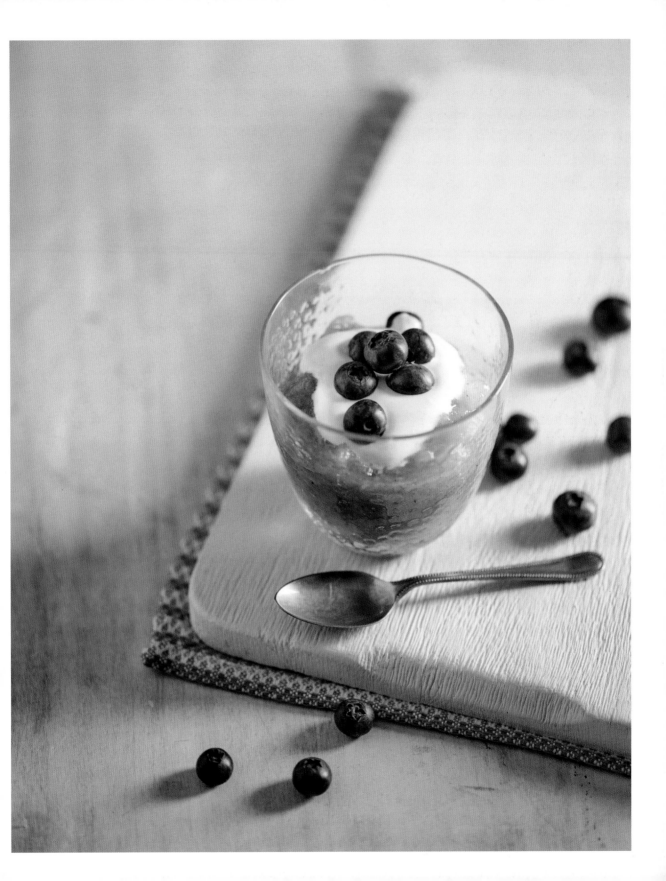

MOVING FORWARDS

Congratulations, you've reached the end of your 21-day plan. Hopefully, you're bursting with health, fizzing with happiness, bubbling with energy – and your tummy isn't doing any of those things; it's just nicely calm and flat.

Now's the time to revisit those measurements and photos you took three weeks ago, and repeat them. Step on the scales, take out the tape measure and see what losses – and gains – you've achieved. Repeat the photographs too, in the same clothes and poses. Bear in mind you might not spot a huge change in these, as it's been a fairly short period for a total-body transformation. But you might be surprised at how even subtle shifts make a difference. It's not just weight or bloating, it's the darkness under your eyes, the colour in your cheeks and the way you hold yourself that may have changed for the better.

Without wanting to sound like TV talent-show judges, remember that this isn't the end of your journey, it's just the beginning. The G Plan is for life and the 21 days is your kick-start. That's why it's a good idea to track measurements and photos, because the chances are that if you record them again in one, two or three months' time, you'll be looking and feeling better still.

So what now?

What happens tomorrow, next week, next month? Well, you have a bank of recipes and ideas to draw on from the past three weeks. Use them, share them, adapt them. Turn to page 128 and you'll find a further collection of tried-and-tested recipes that you can try out. They all still adhere to the G Plan principles. Some are a little more indulgent, others are more practical for packed lunches, while many work for dinner parties or family meals.

What you also have by now are the tools to create your own meals and snacks, based around our guidelines. Now you know how the G Plan works, it's yours to personalize to suit you and your family. But in case you need a crib sheet, here's a reminder:

Vegetables come first. At every meal they should make up at least half of your plate. Try to get into the mindset of planning your meals around what vegetables you have, then adding your meat/fish/other protein as an accompaniment, rather than the other way around. The vegetables are the star.

Add a palm-sized amount of protein, your own palm being proportionate to your needs. Use this as a guideline; it doesn't need to be a grilled chicken breast to work. A hearty serving of lentil soup or a couple of poached eggs work just fine. In other words, don't get hung up on it always having to be meat or fish. Your repertoire now includes plant-based protein, such as tofu, tempeh, pulses and quinoa, as well as eggs and well-chosen dairy. Change it up. Buy meat by all means, but seek good-quality, well-reared meat and buy it less often – we could all do with cutting down on meat for our health as well as the environment.

Add some wholegrains or starchy carbohydrates if you like, but not necessarily at every meal. Don't always revert to obvious choices, such as rice, pasta, bread or potatoes. There are so many grains available: spelt, barley, amaranth, bulgur wheat and millet, to name a few. Even pasta and noodles are available in non-wheat varieties for a change. For an added nutrition boost and to keep things interesting, try sweet potatoes or Jerusalem artichokes when you'd normally have white potatoes. Vary the type of bread you eat: rye, sourdough, spelt or even sprouted. You don't have to spend a fortune on artisan loaves. Wholemeal is the best of the everyday options and wholemeal pitta bread is a budget-friendly standby that's easily stuffed full of interesting salad ingredients.

Keep it real. By avoiding processed foods you automatically avoid most of the ingredients that prevent your microbiome from flourishing. We also recommend the 'is my plate too beige?' test (bread, potatoes, fried food, pastries, pasta, biscuits – all beige). It's a sure sign you need to rebalance your meal to include lots more colourful veg.

The high-diversity diet

This is a truly sustainable healthy eating plan and the most important thing you can do long term is to embrace variety. Avoid having the same breakfast every day, the same common foods at each meal (toast for breakfast, a sandwich for lunch, wheat pasta for dinner), the same few meals on rotation. Always think 'what else could I add?', then throw in some pre- or probiotic extras like nuts, seeds, sprouts, pickles, yogurt – your new gut friends. Try at least one new recipe a week.

Eating seasonally is an excellent way to maintain variety. Pledge to buy a new fruit or vegetable each time you shop, visit local farmers' markets, have a vegetable box delivered or even grow your own. That said, we're also big fans of frozen fruit and vegetables for year-round nutrition, value and convenience.

Cooking from scratch may be the ideal but, of course, there will be times when you need to grab lunch on the go or have a ready-meal for dinner. Don't panic. If there's a choice, go for the product that seems fresher, and has the shorter ingredients list. Then, if possible, tweak it to add nutritional value,

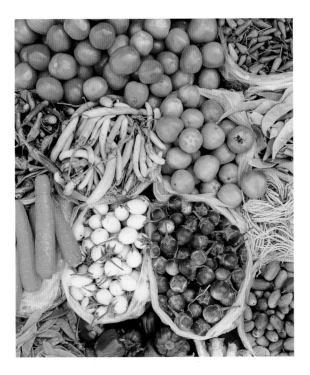

such as adding a bag of salad or ready-chopped microwave vegetables, or opening a can of pulses to add a hit of protein to a ready-made soup.

If you're choosing from café or restaurant foods, your intuition will now inform your best choices (go with your gut feeling!). Avoid the bread, ask for extra veg, sauces on the side, cheeseboard instead of cheesecake... Unless, occasionally, you really, really fancy the cheesecake. Because, above all, we don't want you to feel any fear or guilt around food: Fear of foods you've found don't suit you – yes, they're best avoided but in small amounts they won't kill you. Intolerance isn't a life sentence, it's a guideline. And don't feel guilty if you eat something 'off plan' – everything in moderation is a healthier mindset.

Play by the 80:20 rule

A practical way around these sorts of worries is the 80:20 rule. Eat the G Plan way 80 per cent of the time, but don't stress if 20 per cent of your food isn't perfectly on plan. What does this mean in practice? A good approach is to try always to have a healthy breakfast (it's easier to have nourishing foods to hand at home). Then, of the 14 other meals you'll have over a week, two to three lunches or dinners (but not both) can be a bit more relaxed. That doesn't mean they *have* to be, of course. And it doesn't mean go crazy and have a junk-food feast twice a week for the sake of it. It means don't give yourself a hard time and become a health hermit. Have a social life, give yourself the night off from cooking, relax.

Yes, you can

Don't forget that there are certain foods you might class as indulgent that we now know have a positive effect on our microbiome. Cheese, particularly unpasteurized, is teeming with beneficial microbes, including bacteria, yeasts and fungi, which provide its broad range of distinctive flavours and textures. French scientists have even suggested that cheese microbes could be used to repopulate the microbiome in people taking antibiotics.[25] Dark chocolate, especially if made from raw cacao rather than processed cocoa solids, has been linked to positive changes in the gut. It's a source of polyphenol compounds called flavonoids that have anti-inflammatory, antioxidant actions. And these appear to increase healthy *Lactobacillus* and *Bifidobacterium* bacteria families.[26]

Red wine is rich in a hearty, healthy flavonoid called resveratrol and seems to get the party started for your good bacteria. Data from the British and American Gut Projects shows an increase in microbial diversity in regular alcohol drinkers. A small Spanish study echoed this, finding that daily red wine increased good bacteria and decreased blood lipids (thereby reducing the risk of heart disease).[27] Even coffee keeps the microbiota in balance. It's a surprising source of polyphenols and (unlike tea) some fibre. It has been shown to increase levels of good gut bacteria – so it could be considered a prebiotic drink.[28]

There is, of course, a reason we're only mentioning these small-but-positive benefits now. A diet high in chocolate, wine and cheese isn't likely to get you a Slimmer of the Year award, so for the 21 days they're not encouraged. But now you have the results and resolve to be able to include them in small amounts. So, by all means, enjoy a morning espresso, a couple of squares of good chocolate, a small glass of Merlot and the odd wedge of brie with impunity.

Reflect and refocus

There's a little exercise Amanda does with clients on completing her nutrition and wellbeing retreats and we'd love you to do it too. Switch your phone to selfie mode and take a quick video of yourself, talking about how you feel today. Say what you've lost, how you found the 21 days, how you're feeling physically and emotionally, what the benefits have been. Then make yourself a quick promise about how you're going to hold on to these benefits. That's all, it doesn't need to be long. Then put a note in your calendar for three months' time.

When three months is up, watch your video and remind yourself how great you felt. Hopefully you still do. But if anything's slipped, it provides a good reminder to get back on track.

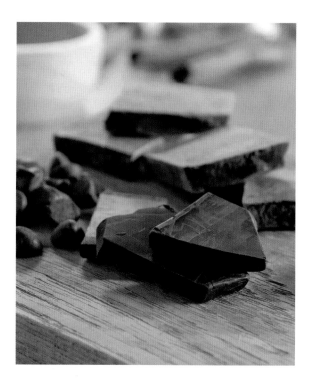

If everything is still good, think about how to keep moving forwards. Start sharing more recipes with your family, helping others to reap the G Plan benefits. Take another video saying how you feel now and what your plans are for the next three months.

If your focus has slipped, use your video to motivate you to get back on track. You could try intermittent fasting if your weight loss has plateaued. Or repeat phases 1 and 2 of the 21-day plan (you don't need to do phase 3 again as you now know the foods you tolerate). Take another video of your intentions and book in another review for three months' time.

The quarterly check-in

In fact, it is a nice idea to repeat phases 1 and 2 of the G Plan every three months, *however* you're feeling. It's always good to give your digestion a rest and remind yourself of all the benefits of home cooking, functional foods and diversity. As the seasons change, spend a fortnight Resting and Re-wilding and you'll feel full of vitality, year round.

We hope you've enjoyed following the 21-day G Plan. Now it's over to you.

WHAT CAN I EAT?

This list is by no means exhaustive, but it can be used as a handy easy-reference guide:

OFTEN (FINE TO HAVE DAILY)

Vegetables

Fruit

Pulses

Unrefined grains, such as quinoa,
  brown rice, oats and spelt

Unsalted raw or soaked nuts

Unsalted seeds (can be toasted)

Eggs (ideally organic)

Pickles

Kefir

Kombucha

Natural yogurt with beneficial cultures
  (dairy options can be increased depending
  on individual tolerance and preference)

Unsweetened non-dairy milk

Herbs and spices

Small amounts of butter (ideally grass-fed)

1–2 cups coffee, green or black tea

A couple of squares of dark chocolate, 70 per cent
  or above

Well-chosen protein, especially oily fish or lean
  organic poultry or fowl, tofu or tempeh

Small amounts of milk (ideally organic, depending
  on tolerance)

A little sea or Himalayan salt

Sweet potatoes

Sea vegetables

Natural coconut water and derivative products

Cold-pressed vegetable oils and coconut oil
  for cooking

SOMETIMES (EVERY FEW DAYS TO WEEKS)

Red meat

Dried fruit (ideally unsulphured)

Dairy products, including cheese, and Greek
  yogurt

Red wine

White rice (basmati, Arborio, sushi, jasmine)

Pasta

Bread

White potatoes

No added sugar soya yogurt

A little natural sweetener for smoothies or
  stirring into porridge or yogurt

RARELY (KEEP TO A MINIMUM BUT NO NEED TO BAN)

Added sugar

Processed foods

Other alcohol

Sugary drinks

MOVING FORWARDS RECIPES

Soups are a great option because you can batch-cook and freeze them in portions for simple evening meals or to take to work for lunch. Serve with oatcakes, toasted rye or sourdough bread, or add some cooked quinoa to the soup for more of a meal.

Roasted Tomato & Chickpea Soup

4 SERVINGS

1kg (2lb 4oz) ripe tomatoes, halved
450g (1lb) cooked or canned chickpeas
4 oregano sprigs, plus extra to garnish
2 teaspoons smoked paprika*
6 garlic* cloves, crushed
2 tablespoons extra virgin olive oil
sea salt flakes
natural yogurt, to serve

Preheat the oven to 180°C (350°F), Gas Mark 4. Place the tomatoes, chickpeas, oregano, paprika and garlic on a baking tray. Drizzle with the olive oil, season to taste and bake for about 1 hour, or until the tomatoes are slightly charred and blackened.

Set aside a few chickpeas to garnish, then transfer the remaining ingredients to a blender or food processor and blend until smooth, adding a little water if necessary to achieve the desired consistency.

Reheat the soup if necessary and serve in bowls with a spoonful of yogurt, a sprinkling of oregano and the reserved chickpeas.

Avocado contains more potassium, which is linked to lowering blood pressure, than a banana. These soups are easy to digest because blending starts the breakdown of the ingredients without losing any of the nutritional or fibre content, meaning they're high in easily absorbable nutrients.

Chilled Avocado Soup

2 SERVINGS

2 ripe avocados
finely grated zest and juice of 1 lemon
½ small shallot
4 dill sprigs, plus extra to garnish
1 handful of fresh coriander
4–8 drops of Tabasco sauce (optional)
sea salt flakes and pepper
250ml (9fl oz) natural yogurt, water or coconut water

TO SERVE:
60g (2¼oz) pumpkin seeds, lightly toasted
natural yogurt (optional)

Scoop the flesh of the avocados into a blender or food processor and add the remaining ingredients. Season to taste and blend until smooth, adding a little cold water if necessary to achieve the desired consistency.

Chill for 30 minutes, if liked, and serve in little bowls, topped with the seeds, a sprig of dill and a small spoonful of yogurt. Eat on the same day to avoid discoloration.

Carrots are easily digested, especially when cooked in soups, plus the ginger and miso are particularly gut-friendly ingredients. Ginger is anti-inflammatory while miso is probiotic and gives a great umami flavour to this soup.

Carrot, Ginger, Miso Soup

2 SERVINGS

1 tablespoon coconut or olive oil
½ onion, chopped
500g (1lb 2oz) carrots, roughly chopped
1 teaspoon fresh ginger* root, peeled and chopped
1 teaspoon miso paste
400ml (14fl oz) just-boiled water
sea salt flakes
1 tablespoon Savoury Nuts & Seeds (*see* page 114), to serve

Heat the oil in a large pan, add the onion and cook for about 8–10 minutes until soft. Add the carrots, ginger and miso paste and stir through for another minute or so before adding the measured water.

Bring to the boil, reduce to a simmer and cook for 10 minutes, or until the carrots are tender.

Blend until smooth using a hand-held blender or a food processor. Check for seasoning, pour into a bowl and serve topped with a scattering of savoury nuts and seeds.

This roast is made with fibrous and prebiotic-rich vegetables to keep your digestion happy and gut bacteria nourished.

Gut-boosting Sunday Roast

4 SERVINGS

½ lemon
1 medium chicken
2 leeks, cut into chunks
3 carrots, cut into chunks
1 red onion, cut into quarters
300g (10½oz) Jerusalem artichokes
   (or new potatoes), halved
olive oil, for drizzling
3 rosemary sprigs, or 2 teaspoons
   dried rosemary
3 thyme sprigs, leaves picked,
   or 2 teaspoons dried thyme
12 asparagus spears, woody ends
   snapped off
1 tablespoon cornflour
200ml (7fl oz) chicken or vegetable
   stock (*see* page 60)
sea salt flakes and pepper

Preheat the oven to 200°C (400°F), Gas Mark 6.

Rub the lemon half over the chicken skin, then place inside the cavity.

Mix all the vegetables, except the asparagus, with the oil, herbs and salt in a large mixing bowl and transfer to a large roasting tin with the chicken. Roast for about 1½ hours, depending on the size of the chicken, until the juices of the leg run clear when pierced with a skewer. Baste two or three times during the cooking period.

Toss the asparagus in a little oil and add to the vegetables for the last 15 minutes.

Remove the chicken from the roasting tin and allow to rest for about 15 minutes before carving. Remove the vegetables and keep warm.

For the gravy, place the cornflour in a small cup with a little cold water and stir until fully dissolved. Place the stock in a small saucepan over a medium heat and bring to the boil.

Slowly trickle the cornflour mixture into the boiling stock, stirring constantly, until it reaches the desired consistency. Season the gravy and serve with the roasted vegetables and chicken.

Beans are a great source of fibre to keep your bowels regular after you finish the programme, while the squash will provide beta-carotene and vitamin A to support your gut lining. Preserved lemons add wonderful flavour to savoury dishes, such as stews and marinades and also to yogurt or dressings. You can use lemon zest and juice if you don't have preserved lemons.

Lemon Cumin Chicken with Smashed Beans

4 SERVINGS

2 garlic* cloves, crushed
2 teaspoons cumin seeds
1 preserved lemon, finely sliced
    (or zest and juice of a lemon)
4 tablespoons natural yogurt
1 tablespoon olive oil
4 chicken thighs with skin
½ butternut squash
2 thyme sprigs, chopped, or
    2 teaspoons dried thyme
200g (7oz) cherry tomatoes
400g (14oz) canned butter beans
    or other white beans, rinsed
    and drained
1 handful of coriander leaves,
    plus extra to serve
1 handful of rocket, plus extra
    to serve
sea salt flakes and pepper

Place the garlic, cumin, lemon, natural yogurt and olive oil in a bowl, add a good pinch of sea salt and mix together. Rub the marinade all over the chicken thighs, cover and set aside in the refrigerator to marinate for about 2 hours.

Remove the seeds from the butternut squash but do not peel it. Cut the flesh into big wedges or half-moon chunks and place in a large roasting tin with the thyme.

Once the chicken has marinated, preheat the oven to 180°C (350°F), Gas Mark 4.

Heat a large frying pan over a high heat and sear the chicken all over until the skin is crisp. Transfer to the roasting tin with the squash, toss together and bake for about 20 minutes. Add the tomatoes and bake for a further 20 minutes until the chicken is cooked through.

Remove the roasting tin from the oven and scatter the beans into the tin, crushing slightly to soak up some of the juices. Cover with foil and leave to rest for 10 minutes to allow the beans to warm through.

Remove the chicken pieces and toss the remaining ingredients together with the coriander and rocket.

Serve the roasted squash and beans with the chicken thighs, topped with more coriander and rocket.

Garlic is an excellent prebiotic with anti-viral properties, so this is a great dish to help rebuild digestion after a stomach bug.

Aromatic Spinach & Garlic Lentils

2 SERVINGS

100g (3½oz) dried red lentils
1 teaspoon ground turmeric
1 tablespoon olive oil
1 onion, sliced
2 garlic* cloves, finely chopped
2 tomatoes, roughly chopped
1 teaspoon ground cumin*
2 handfuls of spinach
juice of ½ lemon

Rinse the lentils in plenty of cold water, then place in a saucepan with twice their volume of water. Add the turmeric and bring to the boil over a medium heat. Cook for about 30 minutes until the lentils are tender, adding a little more water if necessary.

Heat the oil in a small saucepan over a medium heat, add the onion and garlic, then the tomatoes and cumin, and fry for 5 minutes.

Once the lentils are tender, stir in the onion mixture and add a little more water if they are very dry. Add the spinach and set aside for 5 minutes to allow the spinach to wilt and the flavours to infuse. Stir in the lemon juice and serve.

Curry powder is made from a variety of spices, which can help the liver remove toxins from the body and protect against heart disease. Fennel seeds are also traditionally used to relieve bloating and support digestion. This dish is a good way to use up leftover vegetables and is perfect for batch-cooking to be frozen and reheated when you need it. We've served it with natural yogurt for a dose of beneficial bacteria, and brown rice to boost the fibre content.

What's in the Fridge Surprise Curry

2 SERVINGS

1 tablespoon cold-pressed
    rapeseed oil
½ red onion, sliced
1 teaspoon ground cumin*
1 teaspoon curry powder*
1 teaspoon ground turmeric
1 teaspoon fennel seeds
280g (10oz) chicken breast, diced,
    or 200g (7oz) dried red lentils,
    rinsed
360g (12½oz) leftover pulses or
    vegetables, chopped
120ml (4fl oz) coconut milk
1 low-salt vegetable stock cube
200ml (7fl oz) water
juice of 1 lemon
1 tablespoon natural yogurt
75g (2½oz) brown rice, cooked
    according to packet instructions,
    to serve

Heat the oil in a large saucepan over a low heat, add the onion and fry gently for 1 minute. Add the spices and cook for 2–3 minutes to release the flavours.

Add the chicken or lentils, leftover pulses or vegetables, coconut milk, stock cube and measured water, stir well and bring to the boil.

Reduce the heat and simmer, covered, for 15–20 minutes until the chicken or lentils are cooked through.

Stir in the lemon juice and yogurt just before serving the curry on a bed of rice.

Ricotta provides a good dose of protein but is lower in lactose than other cheeses, making it easier to digest. The sweet potatoes are rich in fibre to help keep your bowels regular and support the elimination of toxins. Thyme is a soothing, anti-inflammatory herb that reduces pain and spasms in your gut.

Ricotta, Thyme & Sweet Potato Bake

4 SERVINGS

4 sweet potatoes, scrubbed and cut
 into 1-cm (½-inch) rounds
4 tablespoons cold-pressed
 rapeseed oil
4 garlic* cloves, crushed
3 rosemary sprigs, chopped,
 or 3 teaspoons dried rosemary
2 x 400g (14oz) cans chopped
 tomatoes
2 red onions, thinly sliced
400g (14oz) spinach
400g (14oz) canned butter beans
finely grated zest and juice of
 1 lemon
200g (7oz) ricotta cheese
100g (3½oz) pecorino cheese
3 thyme sprigs, leaves picked,
 or 3 teaspoons dried thyme
sea salt flakes and pepper
green salad or green vegetables,
 to serve

Preheat the oven to 220°C (425°F), Gas Mark 7. Arrange the sweet potato rounds on baking trays in a single layer and drizzle with 1 tablespoon of the oil. Bake for 20–30 minutes until just cooked and starting to brown, then remove the trays and reduce the oven temperature to 200°C (400°F), Gas Mark 6.

Heat another tablespoon of the oil in a saucepan over a low heat, add the garlic and rosemary and cook gently for 30 seconds. Add the tomatoes, bring to the boil, then reduce the heat and simmer for 10 minutes until the sauce begins to reduce and thicken. Season to taste.

Heat another tablespoon of the oil in a saucepan over a low heat, add the onions and cook for 5–10 minutes until softened. Add the spinach and cook until it wilts.

Place the butter beans, with their liquid, in a blender or food processor with the lemon juice and zest and the final tablespoon of oil and blend to make a sauce, adding a little water if it is too thick.

Once everything is ready, layer the ingredients in an ovenproof dish. Start with the tomato sauce, followed by some slices of sweet potato, then the spinach mixture, some ricotta and some white bean sauce and repeat until you've used up all the ingredients. Top with the pecorino and the thyme, then return to the oven and bake for 30 minutes until bubbling.

Serve with a green salad or steamed green vegetables.

TUMMY-FRIENDLY SANDWICHES

We know sandwiches can be helpful when you're out and about. Here are some recipes for simple gut-boosting sandwiches you can prepare and take with you anywhere.

Rye and sourdough breads are better options than plain wheat loaves because they can be more easily digested. They are now widely available in supermarkets but, if possible, try your local baker or farmers' market to get a fresh loaf. It will taste so much better and contain fewer preservatives.

To boost the benefits of a sandwich further, add a spoonful of sauerkraut or kimchi to the filling if possible.

Try some of these ideas for a quick lunch on the go:
- Hummus (*see* page 116), sliced red pepper, rocket and a squeeze of lemon juice
- Smoked salmon, asparagus, shredded spinach and chopped hard-boiled egg
- Avocado, prawns, thinly sliced chilli*, yogurt with lemon zest
- Roast chicken or halloumi, kimchi*, Greek yogurt

NATURALLY SWEET TREATS

These recipes were created for Amanda's signature healthy menu that's served in several five-star spa hotels. They are a little more indulgent than the sweet treats on the 21-day plan, but still contain nutritious and digestion-friendly ingredients.

This dish uses almond milk, but any unsweetened dairy-free milk can be substituted. If you prefer, the chia mixture can be sweetened with a little mashed banana. We serve these pretty little pots with fresh fruit, but chopped dark chocolate makes a great addition, too.

Bramble & Chia Pots

2 SERVINGS

400ml (14fl oz) unsweetened almond milk
50g (1¾oz) chia seeds
seeds scraped from ½ vanilla pod
250g (9oz) fresh or frozen blackberries,
    or other seasonal berries
4 prunes or dates, pitted and finely chopped
fresh fruit, to serve

Place the almond milk, chia seeds and vanilla seeds in a bowl and leave to soak for a few hours or overnight.

Meanwhile, place the berries in a small saucepan over a medium heat with the prunes or dates and a little splash of water. Bring to the boil, then reduce the heat and simmer until the dried fruit has almost dissolved and the sauce has thickened. Leave to cool in the refrigerator.

When ready to serve, divide the chia mixture between two glasses and drizzle with the berry sauce. Serve with your favourite fresh fruit on top.

Dairy-free alternatives can be used instead of the yogurt, but the richness of full-fat dairy makes this a delicious, filling dessert, which is still perfectly healthy. Greek yogurt can also be used.

Fruit can be a tasty and refreshing dessert but not one that always digests easily straight after a meal. Pineapple, however, sits well even after a feast. Thanks to the enzyme bromelain it helps to aid digestion and, partnered with mint, it makes a wonderful palate cleanser.

Orange Blossom & Cardamom Yogurt

2 SERVINGS

250ml (9fl oz) full-fat live natural yogurt
2 teaspoons orange blossom water
2 teaspoons raw honey
seeds from 5 cardamom pods, finely crushed
fresh fruit, to serve

Mix all the ingredients together in a bowl, divide between two serving dishes, top with some fresh fruit and enjoy.

Pineapple Carpaccio with Mint & Lime

3–4 SERVINGS

1 large ripe pineapple
juice of 1 lime
2 tablespoons grated lime zest
6 mint leaves, thinly sliced
1 tablespoon raw honey

Slice the top and bottom off the pineapple and remove the skin and any brown spots. Cut in half lengthways and remove the fibrous centre, then slice the two halves as thinly as possible.

Arrange the pineapple slices on a serving plate and squeeze over the lime juice, scatter the lime zest and mint on top, and drizzle with some honey.

Alternatively, cut the pineapple into slightly thicker slices and cook on a preheated hot griddle pan until lightly charred. Dress as before.

Potassium- and prebiotic-rich banana combines with creamy coconut, a source of medium-chain fatty acids, in this deliciously healthy treat.

Dairy-free Roasted Banana & Coconut Ice Cream

4–6 SERVINGS

3 medium bananas, cut into 1–2-cm (½–¾-inch) pieces
1 tablespoon raw honey
400ml (14fl oz) coconut milk
1 teaspoon vanilla extract
juice of ½ lemon
pinch of sea salt flakes
toasted coconut pieces or raw cacao pieces, to serve

Preheat the oven to 180°C (350°F), Gas Mark 4.

Arrange the banana slices on a baking sheet, drizzle with the honey and toss to coat well. Bake for 30–40 minutes until cooked through.

Scrape the bananas and honey into a blender or food processor and add the coconut milk, vanilla, lemon juice and salt and blend until smooth.

Chill the mixture in the refrigerator until cool, then add to an ice-cream maker or put into a shallow baking tray and place in the freezer, stirring every 20 minutes until it is almost frozen. Leave to freeze for an hour and serve with toasted coconut pieces or raw cacao pieces.

Amanda was first taught this recipe while staying at an Ashram in India – the yoga devotees dreamed up many ways to make the strict vegetarian diet a little bit special. This serves 6–8 people, so make sure you share it!

Chocolate Chickpea Mousse

6–8 SERVINGS

120g (4oz) 70 per cent dark chocolate, roughly chopped
2 tablespoons maple syrup
¼ teaspoon rosewater (optional)
1 x 400g (14oz) can chickpeas (you will only need the liquid from this so use the chickpeas to make a hummus!)
4 teaspoons desiccated coconut, to decorate
12 raspberries, or other berries, to decorate

Melt the chocolate slowly in a heatproof bowl placed over a pan of simmering water and stir in the maple syrup and rosewater, if using. Remove from the heat and allow the chocolate to cool.

Drain the liquid from the chickpeas. Beat the chickpea liquid with an electric whisk or blender until peaks form and you have a fluffy consistency.

Gently fold the melted chocolate into the fluffy chickpea water with a spatula.

Pour the mixture into six small bowls and place in the refrigerator for 30 minutes to set.

Decorate with the desiccated coconut and berries.

The cake you can eat with a good conscience. It provides a source of beneficial fibre and a boost of good fats, courtesy of the creamy avocado.

Avocado & Lime Cheesecake

2 SERVINGS

130g (4½oz) almonds, soaked in
    cold water overnight and drained
50g (1¾oz) desiccated coconut
70g (2½oz) cacao nibs
180g (6oz) pitted dates
3 tablespoons coconut oil, melted
    and at room temperature
dark chocolate, to decorate

TOPPING:
560g (1lb 4½oz) avocado flesh
    (about 5 large avocados)
150ml (¼ pint) lime juice
    (6–8 limes)
175ml (6fl oz) coconut oil, melted
finely grated zest of 5 limes
180g (6oz) agave syrup

Preheat the oven to 150°C (300°F), Gas Mark 2.

Arrange the almonds and coconut on a lined baking sheet and bake for 7–8 minutes until toasted and lightly golden.

Transfer the almonds and coconut to a food processor and add the cacao nibs, dates and coconut oil. Blend until the mixture comes together and is slightly sticky.

Line the base and sides of an 18-cm (7-inch) loose-bottomed cake tin with baking paper and tip in the nut mixture. Press it down firmly with the back of a spoon to form an even layer, ensuring it is neat and flat where it meets the sides of the tin. Chill in the refrigerator while you prepare the topping.

Place all the topping ingredients in a blender or food processor and blend until the mixture is completely smooth and silky. Add a little more lime juice, zest or honey to taste, but keep the mixture tangy.

Pour the topping over the chilled base, cover the tin and return it to the refrigerator for a few hours or overnight until firm.

To serve, carefully remove the cheesecake from the tin and peel off the lining paper. Transfer to a plate and serve immediately, decorated with shavings of dark chocolate or with melted chocolate drizzled over.

RECOMMENDED PRODUCTS

For videos, tips, offers and up-to-date advice on all the latest gut-friendly products, including those you can make yourself at home, and Amanda's 100% Organic Smoothie Booster Kit, visit www.amandahamilton.com.

Unusual ingredients

KEFIR

Kefir and kefir kits can be found in big supermarkets and health-food shops.

KIMCHI AND SAUERKRAUT

Sauerkraut is often available in supermarkets, delis and health-food shops, while kimchi, which originated in Korea is more readily available in specialist delis and Asian supermarkets. You can easily make your own and recipes for both are in a number of books or online. Our favourites are *The Art of Fermentation* by Sandor Ellix Katz and *Pickled* by Freddie Janssen.

KOMBUCHA

Kombucha and home-brewing kits can be found in health-food shops and delis.

MISO

Miso is now widely available in soup sachets or pastes in supermarkets, health-food shops and Asian supermarkets. There are a number of types, including white, red and brown.

FLAXSEEDS, CHIA SEEDS AND PSYLLIUM HUSKS

Flax and chia seeds are now available in some supermarkets and most health-food shops. Psyllium husks will be more readily available in health-food shops and online.

CHICORY ROOT POWDER

This alternative to coffee is available mainly through health-food shops.

GLUTEN-FREE OATS AND OATCAKES

In the UK, Amanda recommends Nairns, available in supermarkets and health-food shops. www.nairns-oatcakes.com

QUINOA

Now widely available in supermarkets and health-food shops. Amanda also recommends Quinoa Crack as a breakfast cereal alternative that's naturally gluten free, available from www.quinoacrack.com

SPECIALIST TEAS

We Are Tea make everyday, tummy-friendly teas, available at www.wearetea.com

SUPPLEMENTS

There are many good-quality food supplements now available. Go for organic choices wherever possible. Amanda recommends Udo's Choice for their Ultimate Oil Blend, Beyond Greens, Super 8 Hi-count Microbiotics and Digestive Enzymes. www.udoschoice.co.uk

RESOURCES & NOTES

1. www.ncbi.nlm.nih.gov/pubmed/21040780
2. gut.bmj.com/content/early/2014/04/29/gutjnl-2013-306541.abstract
3. www.ncbi.nlm.nih.gov/pmc/articles/PMC4757670/
4. www.who.int/dietphysicalactivity/factsheet_adults/en/
5. www.nhs.uk/Conditions/probiotics/Pages/Introduction.aspx
6. www.dailymail.co.uk/news/article-2703772/What-s-dinner-tonight-Lasagne-just-like-week-How-60-people-seven-regular-meals-everyweek.html
7. www.theguardian.com/lifeandstyle/2014/may/14/five-a-day-fruit-vegetables-portion-supermarket
8. jn.nutrition.org/content/early/2016/06/28/jn.115.224683
9. jn.nutrition.org/content/early/2014/12/31/jn.114.199125
10. www.ncbi.nlm.nih.gov/pmc/articles/PMC2683001/
11. www.ncbi.nlm.nih.gov/pubmed/18212291
12. www.ncbi.nlm.nih.gov/pmc/articles/PMC3856475/
13. www.ncbi.nlm.nih.gov/pubmed/18800291
14. www.ncbi.nlm.nih.gov/pubmed/23701561
15. www.cell.com/cell-metabolism/abstract/S1550-4131(15)00389-7
16. www.ncbi.nlm.nih.gov/pubmed/25727903
17. www.thelancet.com/journals/lancet/article/PIIS0140-6736(13)61571-8/abstract
18. www.ncbi.nlm.nih.gov/pubmed/25591978
19. www.ncbi.nlm.nih.gov/pmc/articles/PMC4009525/
20. www.issfal.org/omega-3-fats-may-reduce-risk-of-gastrointestinal-diseases
21. www.ncbi.nlm.nih.gov/pubmed/23518167
22. www.ncbi.nlm.nih.gov/pubmed/21068351
23. www.thelancet.com/journals/lancet/article/PII0140-6736(93)90939-E/abstract
24. www.sciencedaily.com/releases/2009/05/090501162805.htm
25. www.ncbi.nlm.nih.gov/pubmed/17381749
26. www.ncbi.nlm.nih.gov/pubmed/21068351
27. www.ncbi.nlm.nih.gov/pubmed/22552027
28. www.ncbi.nlm.nih.gov/pubmed/29317985

Both imperial and metric measurements have been given in all recipes. Use one set of measurements only.

Eggs should be medium unless otherwise stated. The Department of Health advises that eggs should not be consumed raw. This book contains dishes made with raw or lightly cooked eggs. It is prudent for more vulnerable people such as pregnant and nursing mothers, invalids, the elderly, babies and young children to avoid uncooked or lightly cooked dishes made with eggs. Once prepared these dishes should be kept refrigerated and used promptly.

Fresh herbs should be used unless otherwise stated. If unavailable use dried herbs as an alternative but halve the quantities stated.

Ovens should be preheated to the specific temperature – if using a fan-assisted oven, follow the manufacturer's instructions for adjusting the time and the temperature.

This book includes dishes made with nuts and nut derivatives. It is advisable for readers with known allergic reactions to nuts and nut derivatives and those who may be potentially vulnerable to these allergies, such as pregnant and nursing mothers, invalids, the elderly, babies and children, to avoid dishes made with nuts and nut oils. It is also prudent to check the labels of pre-prepared ingredients for the possible inclusion of nut derivatives.

Vegetarians should look for the 'V' symbol on a cheese to ensure it is made with vegetarian rennet. There are vegetarian forms of Parmesan, feta, Cheddar, Cheshire, Red Leicester, dolcelatte and many goats' cheeses, among others.

INDEX

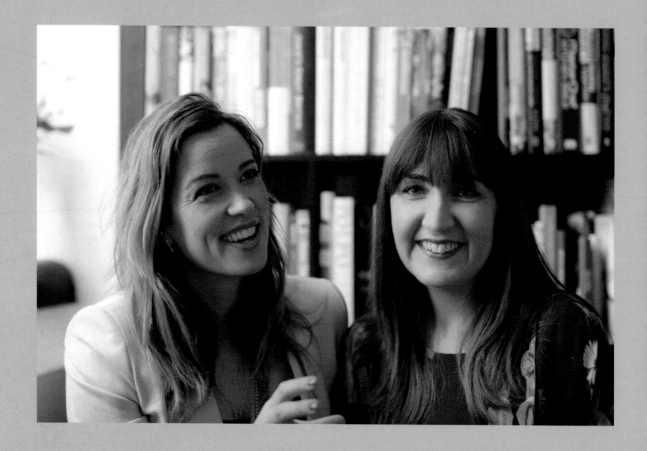

ACKNOWLEDGEMENTS

AMANDA:
Thanks to my back-up team of fellow foodies – Libby, Dina and Beth – helping me to cook up a G Plan storm. To my agents Julia and Jayne, and publisher Kate, whose gut instinct brought this book to life. To Hannah for being a willing guinea pig and awesome co-writer. And to my children Jana and Ruaridh, who are forever my inspiration.

HANNAH:
Thank you Amanda, for your energy and enthusiasm. Your brilliant approach has transformed my eating – and my figure – and I know it will help many others. Kate, it's always a pleasure to work with and learn from you. Wesley, thank you for the book title, you're a genius. And I'm sorry about the state of the kitchen (quinoa everywhere)...